Urological Research

Papers Presented in Honor of William Wallace Scott

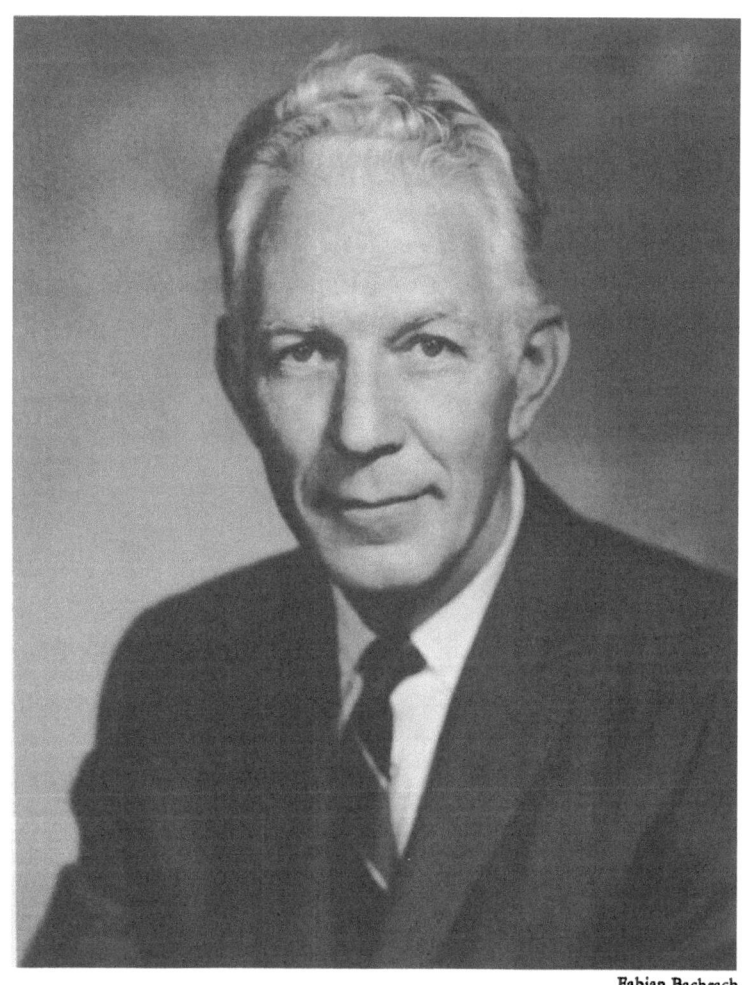

William W. Scott

Urological Research

Papers Presented in Honor of William Wallace Scott

ℙ PLENUM PRESS • NEW YORK–LONDON • 1972

Library of Congress Catalog Card Number 73-179757
ISBN-13: 978-1-4684-1943-6   e-ISBN-13: 978-1-4684-1941-2
DOI: 10.1007/978-1-4684-1941-2

© 1972   Plenum Press, New York
Softcover reprint of the hardcover 1st edition 1972

A Division of Plenum Publishing Corporation
227 West 17th Street, New York, N.Y. 10011

United Kingdom edition published by Plenum Press, London
A Division of Plenum Publishing Company, Ltd.
Davis House (4th Floor), 8 Scrubs Lane, Harlesden, London, NW10 6SE, England

Introduction

Education, patient care, and research combine into the expression of what is known as a university center: a place of learning, a place of development, a place of patient care and cure, a place of compassion, a place of progress. Many centers reflect to the highest degree all of these qualities. Those of us within this volume wish to give testimony to the urological center developed, designed, and cared for by Dr. William Wallace Scott. This man, in our opinion, reflects all of the preceding features to the highest degree. We in Urology have benefited greatly by his leadership and counsel.

Herein will be found articles on patient care, research, education, and historical vignettes. These can hardly be a measure of the man but serve to underline modern progress in Urology and clinical research.

LOWELL R. KING, M. D.
GERALD P. MURPHY, M. D., D. SC.

Patrons

Dr. J. Arcadi

Dr. W. Brannan

Dr. H. Brendler

Dr. H.J. Bradley

Dr. R.W. Bridge

Dr. W.W.S. Butler

Dr. R.L. Calhoun

Dr. W.A. Campbell

Dr. D.M. Davis

Dr. J.N. De Klerk

Dr. R.M. Engel

Dr. R.P. Finney

Dr. R.P. Gibbons

Dr. P.H. Good

Dr. D.A. Goodwin

Dr. Willard E. Goodwin

Dr. J.T. Grayhack

Dr. A.P. Harris

Dr. C.V. Hodges

Dr. J.M. Holland

Dr. W.J. Hopkins

Dr. W.J. Kearns

Dr. L.R. King

Dr. B. Kosto

Dr. A. Mittelman

Dr. G.P. Murphy

Dr. I.J. Nudelman

Dr. L. Persky

Dr. R.B. Roth

Dr. P.L. Scardino

Dr. J.D. Schmidt

Dr. J.H. Semans

Dr. J.W. Smyth

Dr. T.A. Stamey

Dr. H. Schwartz

Dr. W.N. Toole

Dr. J.C. Wade

Dr. K.N. Walton

Dr. Scott's Residents

Brendler, Herbert	April 1946 to January 1947
Doroshow, Herbert S.	January 1947 to July 1947
Hodges, Clarence V.	July 1947 to July 1948
Goodwin, Willard E.	July 1948 to July 1949
Scardino, Peter L.	July 1948 to July 1949
Hudson, Perry B.	July 1949 to July 1950
Bunce, Paul L.	July 1950 to July 1951
Chase, William E.	July 1950 to July 1951
Butler, William W. S., III	July 1951 to July 1952
Ramsom, Charles L.	July 1951 to July 1952
Deklerk, Johan Nico	July 1952 to July 1953
Grayhack, John T.	July 1952 to July 1953
Harris, A. Page	July 1953 to July 1954
Hopkins, William J.	July 1953 to July 1954
Kearns, John W.	July 1954 to July 1955
Arcadi, John A.	July 1954 to July 1955
Stamey, Thomas A.	July 1955 to July 1956
Brannan, William	July 1955 to July 1956
Campbell, William A.	July 1956 to July 1957
Finney, Roy P.	July 1956 to July 1957
Colston, John A. C., Jr.	July 1957 to July 1958
Belt, Bruce G.	July 1957 to July 1958
Burt, Frederick B.	July 1958 to July 1959
Goodwin, Donald A.	July 1960 to June 1961
King, Lowell R.	July 1960 to June 1961
Toole, William Nisbet	July 1960 to June 1961
Bradley, H. John, Jr.	July 1961 to June 1962

Good, Paul H.	July 1961 to June 1962
Schirmer, Horst K. A.	July 1961 to June 1962
Smyth, J. Walter	July 1962 to June 1963
Holland, James	July 1962 to June 1963
Nudelman, Irwin J.	July 1962 to June 1963
Campbell, Edward W., Jr.	July 1963 to June 1964
Mandler, John I.	July 1963 to June 1964
Walton, Kenneth N.	July 1964 to June 1965
Schwentker, Frederic N.	July 1964 to June 1965
Calhoun, Robert E. L.	July 1965 to June 1966
Bridge, Robert W.	July 1965 to June 1966
Gibbons, Robert P.	July 1966 to June 1967
Murphy, Gerald P.	July 1966 to June 1967
Schmidt, Joseph D.	July 1966 to June 1967
Kosto, Bernard	July 1967 to June 1968
Silk, Mark R.	July 1967 to June 1968
Lebowitz, J. Martin	July 1968 to June 1969
Wade, John C.	July 1968 to June 1969
Schwartz, Herbert	July 1969 to June 1970
Engel, Rainer M.	July 1969 to June 1970
Hendricks, Frederick B.	July 1969 to June 1970

Contents

SCIENTIFIC PAPERS

Technology of Induction of Cancer in Rat with Pulse-Doses
of Homogenized Hydrocarbons 3
Charles B. Huggins

Nature and Control of Biochemical Pathways for the Origin
of Prostatic Polyamines............................... 7
H. G. Williams-Ashman

Stilbestrol Antibodies in Prostatic Cancer 21
Mark Silk

Human and Canine Prostatic Metabolism of Testosterone-4-C^{14}.... 25
Menelaos A. Aliapoulios

The Temporal Requirements for Androgens During the Cell
Cycle of the Prostate Gland 27
Michael F. Carter, Leland W. K. Chung, and Donald S. Coffey

Reflections on the Etiology of Benign Prostatic Hypertrophy........ 39
John T. Grayhack

Vesical Suspension in the Management of Obstructive Disease
of the Bladder 51
J. N. DeKlerk

Angiographic Characteristics of Renal Hamartoma................ 61
Herbert Brendler and John W. A. Maguire

Recent Experiences at the Ochsner Clinic with
Transureteroureterostomy 69
William Brannan

The Uses of Intestine in Urology (A "Gut Reaction,"
for W. W. S.)... 75
Williard E. Goodwin

Relocation of Ureteroileostomy Stomata 81
Lester Persky

Technique of Ileal Conduit—Evolution of the Brady Method........ 89
Lowell R. King

Problems in Ileal Conduit Surgery............................. 107
Joseph D. Schmidt

Renal Failure—Remarks on Its Causes 119
David M. Davis

Renin and Erythropoietin Levels in Uremic and Anephric Man 123
Gerald P. Murphy and Edwin A. Mirand

Measurement of Renal Vein Renins or Differential Renal
Function Studies in the Diagnosis of Curable,
Renovascular Hypertension?............................. 131
Thomas A. Stamey

Horseshoe Kidney: Discordance in Monozygotic Twins 151
Elliot Leiter

Renal Metabolism in Obstructive Uropathy 157
Horst K.A. Schirmer

The Nucleosides of Human Urine 161
Arnold Mittelman

Hypospadias: Experience with a One-Stage Repair
(Hodgson Urethroplasty)................................ 169
Rainer M. E. Engel

Rationale for the Use of Nonabsorbable Antibiotics in the
Tseatment of Urinary Infections: Follow-Up Report......... 173
Herbert Schwartz

Vesicoureteral Reflux—Who Needs Ureteroneocystostomy?........ 181
James M. Holland

Studies on the Pathogenesis of Onchocerciasis.................... 189
John. A. C. Colston, Jr.

Recurrent Urethritis in the Female 191
William Nisbet Toole

HIGHLIGHTS

The Brady Urological Institute: Origin, Growth, and Development... 201
  Hugh J. Jewett

Dr. William W. Scott's 25th Anniversary at Johns Hopkins.......... 205
  Clarence Hodges

Reminiscences 209

William W. Scott's First Days at the Brady—A Dialogue 215
  *Peter Scardino, Herbert Brendler, Williard Goodwin,
  and Perry Hudson*

Index 219

Reflections

Sitting here reflecting about my four years (1963–1967) at Johns Hopkins brings many memories to mind:
—The Dome—The Statue
—The Brady Lab—The Brady Library
—Dr. Scott in his long white coat
    The soft voice
    The quiet conservative approach
    The help always given when asked,
        and encouragement when needed
    Residents rounds
    The weekly conference
    X-rays
    The Urological Colloquium
    The birth of a Journal
        and, the making of a Urologist
These are emotional memories
—of work
    pleasure
        satisfaction
            camaraderie
—of gratitude for the opportunity of having
    been part of a great tradition
So in this year of "Nineteen and Seventy-one" *Certain it is* that I am wishing you Dr. Scott a very Happy 25th Anniversary

Robert P. Gibbons, M.D.

SCIENTIFIC ARTICLES

Technology of Induction of Cancer in Rat with Pulse-Doses of Homogenized Hydrocarbons*

Charles B. Huggins†

If you really want to do research, you can do it.
                                                    W. W. Scott

One of the first triumphs of investigative urology was the identification of aromatic hydrocarbons as a cause of cancer. This paper, which is dedicated to William Wallace Scott, relates the story of the unfolding of an epic series of investigations.

The research began with the work of a thoughful and colorful surgeon, Percivall Pott (1713–1788), and his investigation[1] of cancer of the scrotum: "there is a disease as peculiar to a certain set of people, which has not, at least to my knowledge, been publicly noticed; I mean the chimney-sweeper's cancer. It is a disease which always makes its first attack on, and its first appearance in, the inferior part of the scrotum; where it produces a superficial, painful, ragged, ill-looking sore, with hard and rising edges: the trade call it the soot-wart. I never saw it under the age of puberty".

Yamagiwa and Ichikawa[2] discovered that continued simple tar-painting of rabbit ear every 2 or 3 days elicited epithelioma in 32 of 52 ears of surviving rabbits of a strain which never developed spontaneous cancer: "Also unsere Versuchsanordnung war ziemlich einfach. Nur erfordete unser

*This work was supported by grants from the American Cancer Society, The Jane Coffin Childs Memorial Fund for Medical Research, and United States Public Health Service, National Institutes of Health (No. CA 11603).
†The Ben May Laboratory for Cancer Research, University of Chicago, Chicago, Illinois.

Experiment eine aussergewöhnliche Geduld um Jahre und noch länger fortgesetzt zu werden."* It is possible that a factor in the success of the Japanese investigators was proficiency with the brush.

The isolation and identification of carcinogenic hydrocarbons were the work of E. L. Kennaway and his school. The primary discovery[3] of cancer-producing tars arose from pyrolysis of 2-methylbutadiene: "When isoprene is passed through a tube filled with hydrogen and heated to 820 °C a mixture of compounds, chiefly aromatic, is formed; this material produces cancer in mice more rapidly and in a larger percentage of animals than do many samples of coal tar."

The Kennaway school[4] found that the carcinogenic tars exhibited strong fluorescence containing the three-banded spectrum characteristic of benz(a)anthracene. The first pure carcinogenic hydrocarbon to be identified was dibenz(a,h)anthracene; this compound is a weak carcinogen.

During a series of classic investigations of the chemistry of bile acids in 1933, Wieland and Dane[5] isolated a rather strong carcinogenic hydrocarbon, 3-methylcholanthrene, from a natural product, the bile.

The importance of the stoa in the development of the great ideas was known to philosophers in antiquity; often the Arbeitskreis of a laboratory exerts a preeminent influence on the advance of science. In 1937, W. E. Bachmann, a young organic chemist on the faculty of the University of Michigan, was a fellow in the Kennaway school at the Royal Cancer Hospital Research Institute in London. Bachmann and Chemerda[6] in 1938 in Ann Arbor synthesized two new carcinogenic polycyclic aromatic hydrocarbons which are the most powerful of known compounds in the experimental induction of malignant disease.

These compounds are 7,12-dimethylbenz(a)anthracene (7,12-DMBA) and 7,8,12-trimethylbenz(a)anthracene (7,8,12-TMBA). The Bachmann compounds are of critical importance in the evolution of the technology for the rapid induction of cancer in rodents.

Mammary glands of young adult female rats of certain strains are foremost among cells of living creatures in their susceptibility to induction of cancer by irradiation or by hydrocarbons and also in the speed with which the cancers become evident.

We[7] found that a single large but tolerable feeding of any of a number of polynuclear aromatic hydrocarbons or aromatic amines invariably induced mammary cancer in female rats of the Sprague–Dawley (S-D) strain, age 50 days; the first palpable cancer was detected in 20 days after administration of the hydrocarbon, and a considerable proportion of the animals had manifested tumors before the thirtieth day. Of these carcinogens, 7,12-

*[Translation] Therefore, our experimental plan was moderately simple but it demanded extraordinary patience in order to carry it out over many years.

DMBA is more efficient than all others. A single feeding of 7,12-DMBA, 20 mg, dissolved in sesame oil, 1 ml, has elicited mammary cancer in more than 1000 consecutive female rats of S-D strain, age 50–65 days. The superficial position of the mammary gland permits ready detection of the cancers by palpation. The end point is sharp since the cancers are very firm in consistency and discrete. A tumor weighing 8–10 mg can be detected with ease. But subsequent growth of the neoplasm and histological examination are required for confirmation. The high rate of glycolysis (Q_{lac} 12–18) which Warburg found to be an attribute of the metabolism of cancer prevails in the induced mammary cancers[8].

Certain tissues of the rat have a predilection to induction of cancer following the systemic administration of aromatic hydrocarbons. A single meal of 7,12-DMBA provided to 38 rats, observed for 180 days thereafter, evoked tumors as follows: mammary cancer, 100 percent; mammary fibroadenoma, 89 percent; ear duct tumors, two rats; and leukemia, one rat. Tumors of other organs were observed less commonly.

Whereas a single feeding of 7,12-DMBA under the aforementioned conditions always induces breast cancer, intravenous (iv) injection of a concentrated lipid emulsion of 7,12-DMBA is equally effective, less hazardous to laboratory personnel, more convenient, and less costly since smaller doses are required to evoke cancer.

An extensive review of the literature concerning composition and preparation of iv fat emulsions has been published by Geyer[9]. Paul Schurr [10] has devised a method for the preparation of concentrated emulsions of 7,12-DMBA and 7,8,12-TMBA containing 0.5–1 percent (w/w) of the hydrocarbons. These sterile emulsions have a uniform particle size and remarkable stability, persisting more than 3 years.

The LD50 in rat was derived[11] by the probit method after a single iv injection of a lipid emulsion of 7,12-DMBA; the dose causing death of half of the rats was 54 mg/kg.

A single iv injection of homogenized 7,12-DMBA, 13 mg/kg, elicited mammary cancer[12] in 30 consecutive young adult female rats. Stated otherwise, a homogenate of 7,12-DMBA, 2 mg, introduced into the blood as a pulse-dose is not lethal and it is carcinogenic for every rat. In this way an unlimited supply of hormone-dependent carcinomas became available for investigation. The technology of induction is a dependable method which is utterly simple.

REFERENCES

1. Pott, P. Cancer scroti. The chirurgical works of Percivall Pott. London, Wood and Innes, 3:174, 1808.

2. Yamagiwa, K., and Ichikawa, K. Experimentelle Studie über die Pathogenese der Epithelialgeschwülste. *Mitt. Fak. K. Japan. Univ. Tokyo* **15**:295, 1916.

3. Kennaway, E. L. The formation of a cancer-producing substance from Isoprene (2-methyl-butadiene). *J. Path. Bact.* **27**:233, 1924.

4. Cook, J. W., Hieger, I., Kennaway, E. L., and Mayneord, W. V. The production of cancer by pure hydrocarbons. Part I. *Proc. Royal Soc. Lond. Ser. B* **111**:455, 1932.

5. Wieland, H., and Dane, E. Untersuchungen über die Konstitution der Gallensäuren. LII. Über die Haftstelle der Seitenketten. *Z. Physiol. Chem.* **219**:240, 1933.

6. Bachmann, W. E., and Chemerda, J. M. The synthesis of 9,10-dimethyl-1,2-benzanthracene, 9,10-diethyl-1,2-benzanthracene and 5,9,10-trimethyl-1,2-benzanthracene. *J. Am. Chem. Soc.* **60**:1023, 1938.

7. Huggins, C., and Yang, N. C. Induction and extinction of mammary cancer. *Science* **137**:257, 1962.

8. Rees, E. D., and Huggins, C. Steroid influences on respiration, glycolysis and levels of pyridine nucleotide–linked dehydrogenases of experimental mammary cancers. *Cancer Res.* **20**:963, 1960.

9. Geyer, R. P. Parenteral nutrition. *Physiol. Rev.* **40**:150, 1960.

10. Schurr, P. E. Composition and preparation of experimental intravenous fat emulsions. *Cancer Res.* **29**:258, 1969.

11. Huggins, C. B., Ford, E., and Jensen, E. V. Carcinogenic aromatic hydrocarbons: Special vulnerability of rats. *Science* **147**:1153, 1965.

12. Huggins, C., Grand, L., and Fukunishi, R. Aromatic influences on the yields of mammary cancers following administration of 7,12-dimethylbenz(*a*)anthracene. *Proc. Natl. Acad. Sci.* **51**:737, 1964.

Nature and Control of Biochemical Pathways for the Origin of Prostatic Polyamines

H. G. Williams-Ashman*

Feeling greatly honored by this opportunity to join with many other of the admirers, pupils, and friends of William Wallace Scott in paying homage to his outstanding contributions to investigative and clinical urology, I would like to summarize some recent experiments on the biosynthesis of spermine and related amines in the prostate gland and other mammalian tissues. These investigations were initiated during the time I was privileged to serve under Dr. Scott as a staff member of the James Buchanan Brady Urological Institute at Hopkins. The ultimate aim of these studies—to gain insight into the functional roles of the high concentrations of spermine found in the prostate and its secretions in man and certain other mammals—has yet to be achieved. I hope the following paragraphs will show, however, that in delineating for the first time the series of linked enzyme reactions responsible for the production of polyamines in the prostate, a number of novel and previously unsuspected types of biochemical processes have been uncovered, many of which may be of general metabolic significance in nearly all higher animal cells. The findings to be presented were obtained in collaboration with Drs. Anthony Pegg, Dean Lockwood, Juhani Jänne, and Gordon Coppoc.

*The Ben May Laboratory for Cancer Research and Department of Biochemistry, University of Chicago, Chicago, Illinois.

7

Most mammalian cells contain rather small amounts of the diamine putrescine and considerably larger quantities of the polyamines spermidine and spermine. The latter two aliphatic amines contain the elements of putrescine plus a propylamino group ($-CH_2CH_2CH_2NH_2$) attached either to one nitrogen atom (as in spermidine) or to both nitrogen atoms (as in spermine) of the putrescine moiety. The structural formulas of the three bases may be represented as follows, with all of the nitrogen atoms positively charged as a result of addition of protons, as would be expected to occur in the range of physiological pH:

$$\overset{+}{H_3N}(CH_2)_4\overset{+}{N}H_3$$
putrescine

$$\overset{+}{H_3N}(CH_2)_4\overset{+}{N}H_2(CH_2)_3\overset{+}{N}H_3$$
spermidine

$$\overset{+}{H_3N}(CH_2)_3\overset{+}{N}H_2(CH_2)_4\overset{+}{N}H_2(CH_2)_3\overset{+}{N}H_3$$
spermine

As the trivial chemical name "spermine" suggests, this substance was first detected in seminal fluid. In man and certain other mammals whose semens are rich in spermine, the base is found very largely in the seminal plasma rather than in association with spermatozoa, and it originates mainly from the prostate gland. The question as to whether seminal spermine is beneficial to the survival of sperm cells or their transport in the male and female genital tracts, or is in any other way of value to reproductive processes, has been discussed extensively elsewhere[1-4]. The evidence presently available, albeit admittedly quite meager, does not support any of the considerable number of speculations that have been put forward concerning possible reproductive functions of seminal spermine. Although much further work in the latter connection is clearly merited, it is conceivable that the appearance of spermine in prostatic fluid is an epiphenomenon and may simply reflect the washing out of this base, together with other low molecular weight substances, from the cytoplasm of prostatic epithelial cells during the secretory process. Along these lines, it can be imagined that the fundamental physiological importance of spermine and related amines in the male genital tract might relate more to the physiology of the prostate gland itself, and particularly to control of the growth and functional differentiation of the organ by steroid hormones[1-4]. For it is well established that polyamine levels in many mammalian tissues are subject to remarkable changes during periods of rapid growth or differentiation and that these basic substances, which form tight complexes with acid biological macromolecules, can influence profoundly the biosynthesis of DNA, RNA, and proteins[1,3,5,6]. Indeed, Caldarera et al[7]. have hypothesized that androgen-induced alterations in the production of ribonucleic acids in rat prostate may be mediated by changes in the levels of polyamines in this organ. And Moulton and Leonard[8] have postulated that "steroid-induced changes in spermidine levels may play an important role in the synthesis of certain types of RNA, formation of ribosomes, and synthesis of protein in accessory sex organs."

One approach to experimental testing of these hypotheses might be to develop drugs that specifically block the formation of polyamines in mammalian tissues. If this an be accomplished, then it may be possible to stop the accumulation of polyamines in the prostate and its secretions, or in other cells, without interfering directly with other metabolic reactions. This in turn could help to decide whether spermine and spermidine are of central importance for the metabolic economy of the prostate and its hormonal regulation, or for the functions of other animal tissues.

When our investigations were started late in 1967, it was already established that the amino acids L-arginine and L-ornithine could serve as biosynthetic precursors of putrescine in liver and that putrescine and L-methionine provided the building blocks for spermidine and spermine in higher animals[9,10]. But nothing was known about the intermediary enzymic reactions involved in these processes. A major (and perhaps the sole) pathway for the synthesis of spermidine in *Escherichia coli* had already been delineated, however, by the pioneer investigations of Tabor *et al*[11]. published in 1958. These workers demonstrated that the putrescine moiety of spermidine could be formed by the enzymic decarboxylation of L-ornithine. The propylamine portion of spermidine was shown to originate from the carbon chain of L-methionine after loss of the carboxyl group of this amino acid. The latter reaction did not take place with free methionine, but only after it was first converted into *S*-adenosyl methionine (AMe), as catalyzed by the enzyme ATP : L-methionine *S*-adenosyl methionine synthetase. AMe had been discovered some years previously by Cantoni and had been shown to be the methyl group donor involved in many different types of biological transmethylations, as are involved, for example, in the biosynthesis of such diverse substances as epinephrine, creatine, lecithin, and the minor methylated bases present in nucleic acids. The Tabors' finding that *S*-adenosyl methionine could, following enzymic decarboxylation, engage in an entirely different type of group transfer reaction (i.e., propylamino group transfer in spermidine formation) from that occurring in transmethylations was a highly important and revolutionary one from the standpoint of biochemical precedent. Tabor *et al*.[11] further showed that another distinct enzyme (propylamino transferase or spermidine synthase) catalyzed a reaction between the decarboxylated AMe and putrescine to yield spermidine and 5'-methylthioadenosine (MTA). The overall synthesis of spermidine by *E. coli* could thus be accounted for as follows:

$$\text{L-ornithine} \longrightarrow \text{putrescine} + CO_2$$
$$\text{L-methionine} + ATP \longrightarrow AMe + PP_i + P_i$$
$$AMe \longrightarrow \text{decarboxylated } AMe + CO_2$$
$$\text{Decarboxylated } AMe + \text{putrescine} \longrightarrow \text{spermidine} + MTA$$

$$\text{L-ornithine} + \text{L-methionine} + ATP \longrightarrow \text{spermidine} + 2CO_2 + PP_i + P_i + MTA$$

(In these equations, P_i and PP_i refer to inorganic orthophosphate and pyrophosphate respectively.)

We began our studies on the assumption that the synthesis of spermidine in the prostate and other mammalian tissues might proceed by analogous reactions. This proved to be the case, although the details of the intermediary enzymic processes, and especially of the decarboxylation of AMe, turned out to be quite different in animal tissues as compared with *E. coli*. In 1962, on the basis of purely theoretical considerations and without any supportive experimental evidence at hand, the author hypothesized that the biosynthesis of spermine might occur via reactions analogous to those operating in spermidine synthesis, i.e., by a transfer of a propylamino group from decarboxylated AMe to spermidine to form spermine and MTA[1]. Such a reaction does not occur in *E. coli,* which is not at all surprising, considering that *E. coli,* like many other bacteria, neither contains spermine nor is capable of synthesizing it. The prediction that this represented a pathway for spermine synthesis in animal cells was indeed proven experimentally in 1969[12,13].

FORMATION OF PUTRESCINE IN MAMMALIAN TISSUES

A single enzyme appears to be responsible for the production of putrescine in mammalian cells. This is L-ornithine decarboxylase, which is largely if not exclusively localized in the soluble fraction of the cytoplasm. The ornithine decarboxylase of rat ventral prostate[14] and liver[15], is completely specific for the L-isomer of ornithine; the enzyme does not attack related basic substances such as L-arginine and L-lysine, or any other L-amino acids. In this connection, it is noteworthy that it has not been possible to detect any L-arginine decarboxylase activity in higher animal tissues. The latter enzyme is present in a number of bacteria and higher plants. It catalyzes the formation of the base agmatine, the product formed by removal of the carboxyl group of arginine (agmatine bears the same relationship to arginine as putrescine does to ornithine). A number of higher plants and bacteria are also capable of removing the guanido group of agmatine to form putrescine by various enzymic routes, which, together with arginine decarboxylase, provides an alternate pathway for the formation of putrescine. The evolutionary significance of the absence of the agmatine pathway for putrescine production in higher animal tissue is quite obscure.

The ornithine decarboxylase of rat ventral prostate was recently purified to a state of homogeneity[16]. It has a molecular weight of about 70,000. The enzyme requires pyridoxal phosphate as a cofactor. Unlike quite a number of other pyridoxal phosphate–dependent enzymes, the coenzyme of ornithine decarboxylase in prostate and other mammalian tissues readily dissociates from the enzyme; pyridoxal phosphate must therefore always be added to the reaction mixtures used for assay of this enzyme. A peculiar property of the ornithine decarboxylase of animal tissues is that it is very unstable in the absence of low molecular weight dithiol compounds. Decarboxylation of ornithine is powerfully stimulated by dithiothreitol, as well as by other substances containing two sulfhydryl groups such as dihydrolipoic acid or 2,3-dimercaptopropanol. Thiol compounds often employed to activate other sulfhydryl enzymes, such as cysteine or glutathione or 2-mercaptoethanol or coenzyme A, are much less active than dithiols in activating ornithine decarboxylase. A detailed analysis of the loss of activity of the enzyme in the absence of appropriate dithiol compounds[16,17] revealed that prostatic and liver ornithine decarboxylase molecules readily associate into dimeric forms that can be separated by sucrose density gradient ultracentrifugation or by molecular sieving. The dimer of ornithine decarbosylase is totally inactive catalytically in the absence of thiols, but can undergo considerable reactivation in the presence of dithiothreitol, presumably as a result of depolymerization to the protomeric form of the enzyme.

There is a considerable body of evidence that in the nongrowing prostate, liver, and other tissues of adult animals, ornithine decarboxylase may be the least active of the various enzymes responsible for polyamine biosynthesis and that the formation of putrescine may therefore be rate-limiting to the latter. The affinity of ornithine decarboxylase in prostate and liver for its substrate is fairly high; the enzyme exhibits classical Michaelis–Menten kinetics, and the K_m for L-ornithine is about 0.1 mM. The enzyme is inhibited in a competitive fashion by the product of the reaction (putrescine) as well as by the end products of the biosynthetic sequence (spermidine and spermine). The inhibitory constants (K_i) for putrescine, spermidine, and spermine (about 1 mM, 3 mM, and 9 mM, respectively) are sufficiently large, however, that it is debatable whether these inhibitions by the various amines are of physiological importance in living cells[14]. Ornithine decarboxylase appears to be peculiarly insensitive to regulation at a "fine control" level, i.e., by the direct action of small molecules that serve as substrates for neighboring metabolic pathways. The prostatic enzyme, for example, is not influenced by 1 mM concentrations of substances such as AMe, S-adenosyl homocysteine (the product formed when AMe acts as a biological methylating agent), MTA (produced during the synthesis of spermidine and spermine), ATP, and a variety of other nucleotides[16]. On the contrary, ornithine decarboxylase is very readily subject to the "coarse control" type of regulation involving alteration in the levels of the enzyme protein in tissues. The activity of the enzyme in the ventral prostates of castrated rats is, for example, elevated many fold over the first day after injection of androgens[18], and it is increased enormously in rat liver after administration of growth hormone[19] or following partial hepatectomy[20,21], in cultures of chick embryo epidermal cells after stimulation with epidermal growth factor[22], in chick oviduct as a result of estrogenic stimulation[23], as well as in other biological situations. Experiments involving administration of specific inhibitors of ribonucleic acid and protein synthesis strongly suggest that these enormous increases in tissue ornithine decarboxylase are due to enhanced synthesis of the enzyme protein and that in liver the half-life of the enzyme is about 10 min[24]. This is the shortest half-life yet reported for any mammalian enzyme.

DECARBOXYLATION OF S-ADENOSYL METHIONINE IN MAMMALIAN TISSUES AND ITS SPECIFIC ENHANCEMENT BY PUTRESCINE

The enzymic basis of the decarboxylation of AMe in *E. coli* was recently clarified by Wickner *et al.*[25]. They purified the enzyme to a state of homogeneity and showed that it was activated by Mg^{2+} and contained enzyme-bound pyruvate as a prosthetic group. In 1968 Pegg and Williams-Ashman [12] showed that many rat tissues, among which the ventral prostate was by far the most active, contained a soluble enzyme that decarboxylated AMe. In marked contrast to the bacterial AMe decarboxylase, however, the mammalian enzyme did not require Mg^{+2} or any other dissociable metal cofactor but was specifically stimulated by putrescine and to a lesser extent (at saturating amine concentrations) by spermidine. As will be considered shortly, spermidine and spermine are synthesized in mammalian tissues by reactions between decarboxylated AMe and putrescine and spermidine, respectively. The enhancement of AMe decarboxylation by putrescine therefore assumes an especially critical role in the operation of the mammalian multienzyme systems that synthesize spermidine and spermine. For it represents an example of how the product (putrescine) of the first enzyme of a biosynthetic sequence serves as an activator of the second step (AMe decarboxylase) and also as a substrate for the third reaction (spermidine synthase). And putrescine is also a powerful inhibitor of the terminal reaction of polyamine biosynthesis, the spermine synthase reaction[13].

We have recently purified prostatic AMe decarboxylase more than 500-fold and completely separated the protein from the enzymes catalyzing the transfer of propylamino groups from the decarboxylated AMe product that are involved in the production of spermidine and spermine[26]. The nature of the prosthetic group of this mammalian AMe decarboxylase is still unclear. The enzyme is inhibited by certain pyridoxal phosphate antagonists, such as 4-bromo-3-hydroxybenzyloxyamine (NSD-1055)[12]. Depression of AMe decarboxylation by NSD-1055 (which does not inhibit the corresponding bacterial enzyme) is reversed by addition of pyridoxal phosphate, but not by free pyridoxal. These facts would be consistent with the view that mammalian AMe decarboxylase is a pyridoxal phosphate-requiring enzyme(cf. 12). As yet it has not been possible to resolve the enzyme, however, and even the most highly purified preparations are unaffected by pyridoxal phosphate in the absence of antagonists such as NSD-1055[26].

The activation of AMe decarboxylase in prostate and other mammalian tissues by putrescine is dependent on a number of factors. It is increased by lowering the hydrogen ion concentration over the pH range of 5.8–8.7 and by increasing the temperature over the range of 20–45C, and it is dependent on the initial concentration of AMe. In the presence of saturating (2.5 mM) levels of putrescine, the reaction exhibits classical Michaelis–Menten kinetics with respect to AMe concentrations, the K_m for AMe at pH 7.2 and 37C being about 0.05 mM. In the absence of putrescine, the K_m for AMe is appreciably higher than the latter value, and the kinetics of AMe decarboxylation vis-à-vis AMe concentration are complex. These facts hint but do not prove that mammalian AMe decarboxylase is an allosteric enzyme with at least two separate binding sites, one of which interacts with the substrate (AMe) and the other of which, when occupied by the activators putrescine or spermidine, might possibly permit the protein to fold into a configuration that permits more vigorous catalytic activity than observed in the absence of activating amines. Two additional properties of the purified prostatic enzyme are worthy of note in this connection: (a) at saturating levels (5 mM), spermidine activates the decarboxylation of AMe to a much lesser extent than putrescine, and (b) sucrose density gradient ultracentrifugation and gel filtration experiments conducted in the presence of putrescine indicate that the molecular weight of the enzyme is in the same range as that of ornithine decarboxylase (65,000–75,000).

The apparent presence of a specific amine binding site of mammalian AMe decarboxylase that is distinct from the substrate (AMe) binding site holds promise for the development of specific inhibitors of the amine binding site, e.g., congeners of putrescine. Such inhibitors might be expected to depress the formation of spermidine and spermine in vivo without affecting many other reactions in which S-adenosyl methionine is involved, notably a large number of transmethylations.

Activation of carbon dioxide release from AMe by putrescine has been observed with soluble extracts of a wide variety of mammalian tissues other than prostate, including certain malignant tumors. Yet the bacterial enzyme is not enhanced by putrescine but is dependent on Mg^{2+}. This raises the question as to whether putrescine activation of, and lack of magnesium requirement for, AMe decarboxylase is a characteristic of eukaryotic versus prokaryotic cells. Recent unpublished experiments by Dr. G. L. Coppoc negate this hypothesis. The AMe decarboxylase activity of a number of avian and reptilian livers is increased by putrescine but not by Mg^{2+}, and the same findings were obtained with soluble extracts of at least one invertebrate animal tissue, namely, the lobster hepatopancreas. However, an active AMe decarboxylase from another type of eukaryotic tissue, *viz.*, extracts of mung bean shoots, was not enhanced at all by putrescine but, like the *E. coli* enzyme, was dependent on Mg^{2+}. A very active putrescine-activated AMe decarboxylase was found in extracts of baker's yeast; this enzyme did not require Mg^{2+} or other metal ions. On the contrary, the AMe decarboxylase of *Azotobacter vinelindii* is, like the *E. coli* enzyme, a Mg^{2+}-activated protein which is not influenced by addition of putrescine.

ENZYMIC SYNTHESIS OF SPERMIDINE

Rat ventral prostate and liver contain a specific enzyme catalyzing the transfer of a propylamino group from added decarboxylated AMe to putrescine to yield spermidine and MTA[27]. Early attempts[12] to separate this enzyme from putrescine-activated AMe decarboxylase were unfruitful. Recently, however, the enzyme has been purified over 600-fold from rat ventral prostate and completely separated from AMe decarboxylase, and also from another soluble enzyme that catalyzes the synthesis of spermine from decarboxylated AMe and spermidine[27]. By adding purified spermidine synthase to highly refined preparations of AMe decarboxylase, the synthesis of spermidine from AMe and putrescine, readily demonstrable by crude prostatic tissue extracts[12], can be re-established. The Michaelis constant for decarboxylated AMe in the spermidine synthase reaction is not very easy to measure accurately, because of inhibition of the propylamino transfer reaction by high concentrations of substrate (decarboxylated AMe); however, an approximate K_m value for decarboxylated AMe of about 0.01 mM was obtained in recent experiments[28]. Inhibition of the overall reaction by excess decarboxylated AMe is critically dependent on the concentration of the other substrate, i.e., putrescine. These kinetic analyses explain why a stoichiometric formation of spermidine, carbon dioxide, and MTA can be obtained with relatively low overall yields of spermidine when these substrates are incubated with fairly crude prostatic enzyme preparations containing both AMe decarboxylase and spermidine synthase[12]. Up to now, no cofactor for the spermidine synthase reaction has been discovered.

ENZYMIC SYNTHESIS OF SPERMINE

Animal tissues contain an enzyme catalyzing the formation of spermine from decarboxylated *S*-adenosylmethionine and spermidine (spermine synthase). The activity of this enzyme is especially high in soluble extracts of rat ventral prostate and, on a molar basis, is about four times as high as that of the spermidine synthase[13]. Spermidine synthase and spermine synthase can be completely separated from one another. A unique property of the spermine synthase of prostate and liver is that it is inhibited by putrescine, the inhibition being competitive with respect to spermidine[13]. It is interesting that the K_i for putrescine inhibition of the spermine synthase reaction has about the same value (0.1 mM) as the K_m for putrescine as an activator of AMe decarboxylase in rat prostate. This suggests that the intracellular levels of putrescine may play a key role in regulation of the synthesis of spermidine versus spermine. These observations also are in line with the report of Raina and Hannonen[29] that various preparations obtained by ammonium sulfate fractionation of regenerating rat exhibit constancy in the ratio of their activities in promoting spermidine and spermine synthesis from AMe as compared with decarboxylated AMe and also that very low levels (0.02 mM) of putrescine evoked small increases in spermine synthesis from AMe, but not from decarboxylated AMe. The latter finding fits in well with the enhancement of mammalian AMe decarboxylation by putrescine. As is the case with spermidine synthase, there is no evidence available to indicate that spermine synthase contains a prosthetic group.

FATE OF 5'-METHYLTHIOADENOSINE

The foregoing indicates that MTA is a product of the synthesis of both spermidine and spermine by the enzymic reactions described. Accumulation of MTA as a result of polyamine formation would be expected to deplete the pool of adenine nucleotides in tissues, since AMe and decarboxylated AMe are ultimately derived from ATP. We therefore examined mammalian tissues for enzymes that might degrade MTA. Such an enzyme was found to be highly active in soluble extracts of rat ventral prostate. It catalyzes the formation of free adenine from MTA, and once the enzyme is partially purified, it exhibits an absolute requirement for P_i. The available evidence suggests[30] that this MTA-degrading enzyme catalyzes the following reaction:

$$MTA + P_i \longrightarrow adenine + 5\text{-methylthioribose-1-phosphate}$$

As might be expected, P_i can be replaced by inorganic arsenate in this reaction. The phosphate-dependent MTA-splitting enzyme is not identical with any known mammalian purine nucleoside phosphorylase[30]. Prostatic phosphatases apparently can split 5-methylthioribose-1-phosphate to yield P_i and 5-methylthioribose. The biological fate of the latter sulfur-containing sugar is completely obscure and is worthy of experimental scrutiny. The operation of the enzyme promoting phosphorolytic cleavage of MTA *in vivo* would serve to drag the reactions involved in spermidine and spermine biosynthesis to completion and to prevent extensive accumulation of MTA in tissues.

METHIONINE ANALOGUES AND POLYAMINE BIOSYNTHESIS

Certain analogues of methionine are known to serve as substrates for mammalian AMe synthetases, resulting in the formation of the corresponding analogues of AMe. One of the analogues of methionine that has been the subject of intensive investigation in this respect is ethionine, in which the methyl group of methionine is replaced by an ethyl group. Administration of ethionine results in profound changes in liver metabolism, and in some species the analogue is carcinogenic after prolonged feeding. Many of the toxic actions of ethionine are thought to be due to the gross decline in tissue ATP levels, especially in liver, that are a concomitant of the synthesis of *S*-adenosyl ethionine (AEt) *in vivo*[31]. Despite the fact that AEt can ethylate a number of cellular constituents as a result of its utilization by certain transmethylating enzymes, the rates of reaction from the ethyl analogue are often much slower than from AMe, so that AEt accumulates and the total tissue ATP is serverely depleted. The precursor function of AMe in polyamine synthesis as well as in many transmethylation reactions made it of considerable interest to examine the possible participation of AEt in the biosynthesis of spermidine and spermine. It was found by Pegg[31] in the author's laboratory that AEt is only slowly decarboxylated by prostatic AMe decarboxylase, although carbon dioxide release was enhanced by putrescine and spermidine in a manner similar to that observed with the more active natural AMe substrate. The rates of spermidine production from AEt and putrescine, and of spermine formation from AEt and spermidine, by crude prostatic enzyme preparations were also much lower than that observed with AMe as the ultimate propylamino group donor. Thus AEt is only feebly active as a precursor of polyamines, and it was additionally shown that AEt inhibits the formation of spermidine from AMe and putrescine[31]. These results suggest that ethionine administration might cause a fall in tissue polyamine levels, and it has indeed been reported that spermine and spermidine concentrations in liver fall after ethionine treatment of the animals[32], although on continued administration of ethionine, hepatic spermidine levels gradually return to normal. It seems improbable that the very low rate of formation of spermidine from AEt could account for the latter phenomenon, and this further indicates that alternate pathways for spermidine and spermine may occur in animal cells. One such possible reaction would be a dismutation between two molecules of spermidine:

$$2 \text{ spermidine} \rightleftharpoons \text{spermine} + \text{putrescine}$$

Elsewhere[3], a plea has been entered that a lookout be kept for this reaction in mammalian tissues.

POLYAMINES AND THEIR ENZYMIC SYNTHESIS DURING REGRESSION AND GROWTH OF THE PROSTATE

The ventral prostates of normal adult rats contain about 6 μmoles each of spermidine and spermine per gram fresh weight of tissue and much lower amounts of putrescine (about 0.3 μmoles per gram). These values include polyamines present both in various cell types in the gland and in the secretions stored in the lumina. After orchiectomy there occurs a marked decline in the total putrescine and spermidine levels. The content of spermine also falls as a result of androgen withdrawal, although more slowly than in comparison with spermidine[18]. When rats that had been castrated 1 week previously were given large daily doses of testosterone, there was a very significant increase in ventral prostate putrescine and spermidine levels within 24 hr and restoration to normal values within 5 days or so. The spermine concentrations under the same conditions rose much more slowly and were not elevated significantly until the fifth day after commencement of daily androgen injections. Prostatic ornithine decarboxylase and putrescine-dependent AMe decarboxylase activities were also diminished immensely after orchiectomy, declining to 15% and 7% of the norm within 7 days after removal of the testes. Following subsequent daily administration of testosterone, ornithine decarboxylase and AMe decarboxylase activities doubled within 6 and 3 hr, respectively, and were increased fourfold and tenfold within 2 days after starting the hormone treatments. Thus it was evident that during the early phases of androgen-induced growth of rat ventral prostate, increased accumulation of putrescine and spermidine can occur *pari passu* with enhanced activities of the two key decarboxylating enzymes. However, consideration of the chronology of these changes in spermidine levels *vis-à-vis* early androgen-dependent enhancement of nuclear RNA synthesis in the prostate provides no compelling reasons to believe that spermidine and spermine are mediators of the effects of androgens on the genetically determined RNA- and protein-synthesizing apparatus of this gland. Rather it would appear that a coupling between RNA formation on the one hand, and spermidine synthesis on the other, takes place during the early stages of androgen-induced prostatic growth. The functional significance of this may be that spermidine is of considerable importance in neutralizing the large excess of negative charges that occurs intracellularly as a result of a greatly increased accumulation of ribonucleic acids, in bulk in the form of cytoplasmic polyribosomes.

L'ENVOI

These studies indicate that the polyamines spermidine and spermine are formed in the prostate and other mammalian tissues from the amino acids L-ornithine and L-methionine. Ornithine has never been found to occur in animal proteins but is readily formed from the amino acid L-arginine by the action of the enzyme arginase. It has been known for a long time that the livers of animals that excrete urea as their major end product of nitrogen metabolism are rich in arginase, the formation of urea being very largely confined to the liver. Yet many extrahepatic tissues, including the prostate gland[3], contain arginase, even though they cannot synthesize urea from carbon dioxide and ammonia or various amino acids. The presence of arginase in extrahepatic tissues has long been an enigma, but now it seems reasonable to postulate that the function of this enzyme in tissues that cannot carry out the complete urea cycle is to provide ornithine for the synthesis of putrescine, and hence of both spermidine and spermine[3].

The widespread occurrence of spermidine and spermine among higher animal tissues, and the exceedingly high concentrations of spermine in the prostate secretion of some mammalian species, still remains very much of a puzzle. Presumably, the formation of these polyamines, which serves to remove the key amino acids methionine and arginine from their utilization in the synthesis of proteins and also in the synthesis of small molecules such as creatine and many other methylated tissue constituents, cannot be entirely useless or vestigial. For one would think, if the latter were the case, that the enzymes necessary for polyamine formation would have been lost in many instances by a process of natural selection during the complex evolution of higher animal organisms. The possibility that spermidine and spermine play an important role as intracellular regulators of nucleic acid and protein synthesis is, as considered above, an attractive one. However, unequivocal evidence in support of such functions of polyamines in mammalian tissues is still lacking, despite a variety of experimental hints in this direction. Now that the enzymes for at least one of the major pathways for the biosynthesis of spermidine and spermine have been isolated and characterized, it may not be totally unreasonable to hope that specific inhibitors of one of more of these catalysts may be discovered in the not too far distant future. Application of these inhibitors to living animals so as to block polyamine formation in various tissues may then help to decide whether polyamines are indeed essentially regulators of macromolecular biosynthetic or other important metabolic processes and might also cast light on the mysterious role, if any, of the large amounts of spermine found in prostatic secretions.

The author is very deeply grateful to William Wallace Scott for the wonderful and unfailing support he gave to these and other ivory tower biochemical investigations, and to the author and his biochemist colleagues, throughout the happy years he worked in the Brady Laboratory for Reproductive Biology.

REFERENCES

1. Williams-Ashman, H. G. In *On Cancer and Hormones: Essays in Experimental Biology*, pp. 325–346, (1962).
2. Williams-Ashman, H. G. *Invest. Urol.* 2:605, 1965.
3. Williams-Ashman, H. G., Pegg, A. E., and Lockwood, D. H. *Advan. Enzyme Regulation* 7:291, 1969.
4. Williams-Ashman, H. G., and Lockwood, D. H. *Ann N. Y. Acad. Sci.* 171:882, 1970.
5. Tabor, H., and Tabor, C. W. *Physiol. Rev.* 16:245, 1964.
6. Herbst, E. J., and Bachrach, U. (eds.) *Metabolism and biological functions of polyamines.* *Ann. N.Y. Acad. Sci.* 171:691–1009, 1970.
7. Caldarera, C. M., Moruzzi, M. S., Barbiroli, B., and Moruzzi, G. *Biochem. Biophys. Res. Commun.* 33:266, 1968.
8. Moulton, B. C., and Leonard, S. L. *Endocrinology* 84:1461, 1969.
9. Jänne, J. *Acta Physiol. Scand. Suppl.* 300:1, 1967.
10. Siimes, M. *Acta Physiol. Scand. Suppl.* 298:1, 1967
11. Tabor, H., Rosenthal, S. M., and Tabor, C. W. *J. Biol. Chem.* 233:907, 1958.
12. Pegg, A.E., and Williams-Ashman, H. G. *J. Biol. Chem.* 244:682, 1969
13. Pegg, A.E., and Williams-Ashman, H. G. *Arch. Biochem. Bipohys.* 137:156, 1970.
14. Pegg, A.E., and Williams-Ashman, H. G. *Biochem J.* 108:533, 1968.
15. Jänne, J., and Raina, A. *Acta Chem. Scand.* 22:1349, 1968.
16. Jänne, J., and Williams-Ashman, H. G. *J. Biol. Chem.* 246:1725, 1971.
17. Jänne, J., and Williams-Ashman, H. G. *Biochem. J.* 119:595, 1970.
18. Pegg, A.E., Lockwood, D. H., and Williams-Ashman, H. G. *Biochem. J.* 117:17, 1970.
19. Jänne, J., Raina, A., and Siimes, M. *Biochim. Biophys. Acta* 166:419, 1968.
20. Russell, D. H., and Snyder, S. H. *Proc. Natl. Acad. Sci.* 60:1420, 1968.
21. Schrock, T.R., Oakman, N.J., and Bucher, N. L. R. *Biochim. Biophys. Acta* 204:564, 1970.
22. Stastny, M., and Cohen S. *Biochim. Biophys. Acta* 204:578, 1970.
23. Cohen, S., O'Malley, B. W., and Stastny, M. *Science* 170:336, 1970.
24. Synder, S.H., Kreuz, D. S., Medina, V. J., and Russell, D. H. *Ann N.Y. Acad. Sci.* 171:749, 1970.

25. Wickner, R. B., Tabor, C. W., and Tabor, H. *J. Biol. Chem.* **245**:2132, 1970.
26. Jänne, J., and Williams-Ashman, H. G. *Biochem. Biophys. Res. Commun.* **42**:222, 1971.
27. Jänne, J., Schenone, A., and Williams-Ashman, H. G. *Biochem. Biophys. Res. Commun.* **42**:758, 1971.
28. Jänne, J., and Williams-Ashman, H. G. Unpublished observations.
29. Raina, A., and Hannonen, P. *Acta Chem. Scand.* **24**:3061, 1970.
30. Pegg, A.E., and Williams-Ashman, H. G. *Biochem. J.* **115**:241, 1969.
31. Pegg, A.E. *Biochim. Biophys. Acta* **177**:261, 1969.
32. Raina, A., Jänne, J., and Siimes, M. *Acta Chem. Scand.* **18**:1804, 1964.

Stilbestrol Antibodies in Prostatic Cancer

Mark Silk*

I would like to join with the other "Bradyites" to extend my thanks and congratulations to Dr. Scott on this, the twenty-fifth year of his chairmanship of the Department of Urology at the Johns Hopkins Hospital. Under Dr. Scott's tutelage I have learned all I know about urology. My present limited knowledge is due to no fault on his part but results from my forgetting most of the things he has taught me. But the one thing I will never forget is how to show Dr. Scott's Tuesday and Thursday morning private clinic patients "where the toilet paper is and how to use sink."

From the beginning of my urological residency I can recall Dr. Scott's aversion to the routine maintenance of patients with prostatic carcinoma on diethylstilbestrol without specific indications. Subsequent studies by the Veterans Administration Cooperative Study Group have verified his earlier conclusions. This study suggests one additional possible difficulty that may be encountered in long-term diethylstilbestrol therapy.

Anti-insulin antibodies have been demonstrated in man. They have been shown experimentally and clinically to be of importance in the development of insulin-resistant diabetes mellitus[1]. Many patients with prostatic carcinoma develop an unresponsiveness to diethylstilbestrol (DES)[2]. This may be the result of tumor unresponsiveness secondary to progressive cellular undifferentiation. However, in some of these patients a remission

*University of Connecticut Medical School, Department of Urology, Hartford, Connecticut.

can be brought about by simply altering the type of estrogen compound being administered([2,3]). This remission is often accomplished with estrogen dosages that are equivalent to, or less than, that of the original diethylstilbestrol dosage. Although this may represent changes in tumor metabolism and physiology, this study was undertaken to attempt to demonstrate a humoral factor, antidiethylstilbestrol antibodies, which may in part account for these clinical observations.

METHOD

Serum was obtained from ten healthy male volunteers who had never received diethylstilbestrol and from 20 men with prostatic carcinoma who had been maintained on diethylstilbestrol, 1 mg/tid, for a minimum of 180 days. The serum was incubated with labeled diethylstilbestrol-H^3 at 37°C and subjected to paper electrophoresis. The electrophoretic pattern was identified and divided, and the radioactivity was determined with a liquid scintillation counter.

RESULTS

Controls

There were two peaks of radioactivity obtained when DES was added to normal plasma. One migrated with β-globulin and the other with albumin (Fig 1).

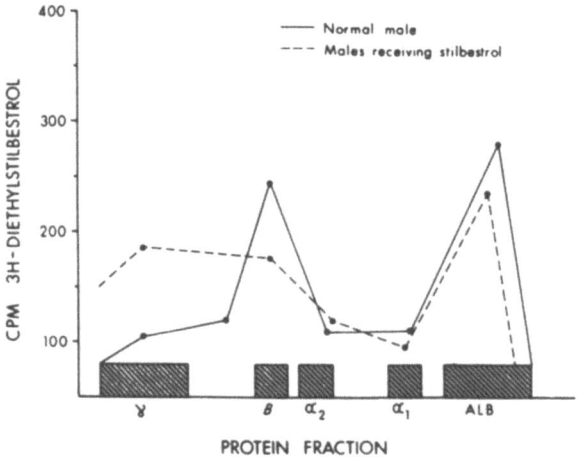

Fig. 1.

Experimental

In addition to the two peaks (BG and alb) noted in the controls, 13 of the 20 patients who were receiving DES had an additional peak of radioactivity that migrated with γ-globulin (Fig. 1).

DISCUSSION

When human plasma has been incubated with a number of labeled gonadal steroids and subjected to paper electrophoresis, peaks of radioactivity can be demonstrated at the albumin and β-globulin sites[4]. Several authors have demonstrated the presence of a gonadal steroid globulin (GBG) in human plasma that migrates with β-globulin. The amount of labeled gonadal steroid bound at this site varies with the specific compound, prior loading with stable compounds, and the sex and age of the individual[5,6]. Diethylstilbestrol has a relatively low affinity for GBG compared to testosterone and estradiol. Our studies with normal plasma confirm these prior observations.

In addition, we were able to demonstrate labeled DES migrating with γ-globulin in men who had previously received DES. Experimentally, prior plasma loading with stable gonadal steroid compounds, which may be considered equivalent to a patient receiving gonadal steroids, resulted in migration of labeled gonadal steroids with inter α-globulin[4]. This is presumed to be secondary to saturation of the binding sites on GBG. In those studies, none of the labeled compounds migrated with γ-globulin. Binding of a compound and migration with γ-globulin are accepted by most investigators as a nonspecific indication of antibody formation[7]. For example, the initial observation of migration of labeled insulin with γ-globulin has been subsequently demonstrated by methods of antibody purification to be a manifestation of antibody formation[1]. The migration of labeled DES with γ-globulin in patients who had previously received DES strongly suggests the presence of anti-DES antibodies in these patients.

DES is a nonprotein steroidal compound. When antibodies are formed against nonprotein-containing substances, the antigen behaves as a haptene. An antibody that is produced against a nonprotein substance and a protein component will react to the nonprotein substance alone, to the protein, or to the conjugated protein[7]. The exact identification of a DES antibody awaits further specific purification, definition, and quantification.

The serum studied was obtained from a population of patients with prostatic carcinoma who were receiving DES. Unfortunately, these patients were lost to follow-up and no correlation can be made between the presence of antibodies and the clinical status of these patients. Our present studies will attempt to better delineate this antibody and its possible relationship to the progression of disease in patients with prostatic carcinoma.

REFERENCES

1. Williams, R. H. The pancreas. In *Textbook of Endocrinology,* Williams, R. H. (ed.), W.B. Saunders Company, Philadelphia, 1968.
2. Desberg, D. Advanced prostatic carcinoma: Alteration of estrogen therapy. *J. Urol.* **83**:461, 1960.
3. Morales, P. A., Brendler, H., and Hotchkiss, R. Role of the adrenal cortex in prostatic carcinoma. *J. Urol.* **73**:399, 1955.
4. Rosner, W. Interaction of adrenal and gonadal steroids with proteins in human plasma. *New Engl. J. Med.* **281**:658, 1969.
5. Rosner, W., and Deakins, S. M. Testosterone binding globulins in human plasma: Studies on sex distribution and specificity. *J. Clin. Invest.* **47**:2109, 1968.
6. Vermeulen, A., and Verdonck, L. Studies on the binding of testosterone to human plasma. *Steroids* **11**:609, 1968.
7. Campbell, D., Garvey, J. S., Cremer, N.E., and Sussdorf, D. H. (eds.), *Immunology,* W. A. Benjamin, Inc., New York, 1964.

Human and Canine Prostatic Metabolism of Testosterone-4-C^{14}

Menelaos A. Aliapoulios*

It first became obvious in my student days at Johns Hopkins Medical School that the prostate gland, guardian of the outlet of the urological system, served a very vital and important function. In addition, it is of interest that the dog is the only species which shares with man an age-dependent tendency to develop benign prostatic hyperplasia and adenocarcinoma of the prostate. Under the stimulus of Dr. W. W. Scott and Dr. Fred Burt at the Brady Institute, methods were mastered for the analysis of steroid hormones in urine of normal subjects as well as prostatic cancer patients. These studies were later continued and embellished in collaboration with Dr. Peter Ofner at the Steroid Biochemistry Laboratory of the Medical Services, Lemuel Shattuck Hospital, and in the Departments of Pharmacology and Surgery, Harvard Medical School, Boston, Massachusetts.

It has become apparent from the study of excretory end-products of testosterone metabolism in normal subjects and patients with gonadal dysfunction syndromes that target tissues for male hormone action are the chief contributors to the pool of 5α-androstane-3α,17β-diol glucuronide and that determination of this urinary steroid provides a measure of male sexual differentiation. The mechanism of androgen action therefore appears intimately related to the metabolism of circulating C$_{19}$-steroids at the target site.

We have studied comparative androgen metabolism in the canine and human prostate with respect to (a) various aspects of testosterone and

*Chief of Surgery, Cambridge Hospital, Cambridge, Massachusetts, and Assistant Professor of Surgery, Harvard Medical School, Boston, Massachusetts.

5α-dihydrotestosterone transformation by prostatic tissue preparations, (b) properties of the prostatic enzymes responsible for the formation of 5α-dihydrotestosterone, 5α-androstane-3α,17β-diol, and 5α-androstane-3β, 17β-diol, and (c) the fate of testosterone-4-C^{14} in the canine prostate and urinary bladder as well as the human prostate.

Physiological amounts of testosterone-4-C^{14} were infused into the common arterial supply of the prostate gland and urinary bladder of five adult dogs and two human subjects. Only the labeled hormone was found in blood from the inferior vena cava 2 min after the beginning of the infusion until the dog was sacrificed 9 min later. Uptakes by prostate and urinary bladder accounted for 1–5 % and 0.9–3 %, respectively, of the substrate radioactivity. Metabolism of the infused testosterone-4-C^{14} in the canine and human prostate was extensive and yielded, almost exclusively, 5α-reduced products. There was a several-fold predominance of 17β-hydroxy metabolites over the 17-ketone analogues and of 3β-hydroxy metabolites over the 3α-epimers. Half of the prostate radioactivity was associated with two major transformation products, 5α-dihydrotestosterone (17β-hydroxy-5α-androstan-3-one) and 5α-androstane-3β,17β-diol. In contrast, metabolism of testosterone-4-C^{14} in the urinary bladder was much more limited and oxidative, with 4-androstane-3,17-dione as the major and 5α-androstane-3,17-dione as the minor products. The different pathways of male hormone metabolism in tissues which have a common embryonic origin, yet are unlike in their response to androgen, and the identification of twomajor prostate metabolites with distinct biological modes of action suggest that testosterone-5α-reductase and 3β-hydroxy-C^{19}-steroid oxidoreductase are systems which regulate androgenic activity at the target site.

Results of these studies are related to evidence that the 5α-reduced 17β-hydroxysteroid metabolites affect androgen action at the target site.

The Temporal Requirements for Androgens During the Cell Cycle of the Prostate Gland

Michael F. Carter,* Leland W. K. Chung,* and Donald S. Coffey*

PERSPECTIVE

Dr. William Wallace Scott has focused a considerable portion of his efforts toward defining the clinical parameters and physiological factors which are important in understanding and controlling the growth of the prostate gland. Dr. Scott defined the ultimate clinical goal in his statement, "What a glorious day it will be for urology when we can shrink the benign nodular hyperplastic prostate, quiet the carcinomatous one and increase the libido and potentia all with a tablet. Oh happy day!"[1] Dr. Scott has initiated this long and difficult journey through a series of contributions which have formed a systematic framework for the evaluation and search for new inhibitors of prostatic growth[1-18]. This has been exemplified by his leadership in the recent development of antiandrogenic drugs, which introduce a great deal of promise as a new approach for the effective treatment of benign nodular prostatic hyperplasia and prostatic carcinoma[12,14,17,18].

Antiandrogens are a unique group of compounds by virtue of their essential absence of estrogenic properties and their ability to directly displace androgens from target organs such as the prostate and seminal vesicles. In November 1963, Dr. Scott initiated studies on a new oral progestational steroid with strong antiandrogenic properties. This compound, SH-714, was produced by Schering A.G. Berlin, under the generic name of cypro-

*The James Buchanan Brady Urological Institute and the Department of Pharmacology and Experimental Therapeutics, The Johns Hopkins Hospital, Baltimore, Maryland.

terone acetate or 6-chloro-$\Delta^{4,6}$-pregandiene-17-ol-3,20-dione-17-acetate. This drug is strongly progestational (250 times more active than progesterone), weakly estrogenic (1/1000 times as active as estradiol), and weakly androgenic (1/640 as active as testosterone propionate). When cyproterone acetate is administered to normal male dogs or rats, there is a marked decrease in prostatic size and function[14,17]. Dr. Scott extended these laboratory observations by introducing clinical trials with cyproterone acetate on patients with prostatic cancer and benign prostatic hyperplasia[17,18]. The clinical results have been most promising, and it appears that these new antiandrogen drugs may provide a new therapeutic approach to the urologist. The current usages of estrogens are sometimes associated with painful enlargement of the breast and loss of libido and may be contraindicated in certain forms of cardiovascular disease. However, these do not appear to be serious limitations with the clinical use of antiandrogens. At present, several new antiandrogens are being evaluated, and it is anticipated that those drugs will soon find an important place in the treatment of abnormal prostatic growth.

In addition to the clinical importance of antiandrogens, they also provide a powerful experimental tool in elucidating the role of androgens in the growth of the prostate gland. For example, in the accompanying paper, use of cyproterone acetate as a chemical probe to competitively displace testosterone from the rat ventral prostate gland is described. This procedure permits one to ascertain the temporal requirements of testosterone in the prostate for the initiation of DNA synthesis and cell division.

A more precise insight into the regulation of DNA synthesis in the prostate is required because this represents the uncontrolled component producing the hyperplastic element in the abnormal growth of the human prostate.

A SELECTED BIBLIOGRAPHY (1955–1970) OF CONTRIBUTIONS BY DR. WILLIAM WALLACE SCOTT PERTAINING TO EXPERIMENTAL STUDIES ON PROSTATIC GROWTH

1. Scott, W. W., Hopkins, W. J., Lucas, W. M., and Tesar, C. A search for Inhibitors of prostatic growth stimulators. *J. Urol.* **77**:652, 1957,
2. Grayhack, J. T., Bunce, P. L., Kearns, J. W., and Scott, W. W. Influence of the pituitary on prostatic response to androgens in the rat. *Bull. Johns Hopkins Hosp.* **96**:154, 1955.
3. Scott, W. W. Regulators of prostatic growth. *Trans. Am. Assoc. Genitourin. Surg.* **58**:168, 1956.
4. Burt, F. B., Finney, R. P., and Scott, W. W. Steroid response to therapy in prostatic cancer. *J. Urol.* **77**:485, 1957.
5. Goodwin, D. A., Rasmussen-Taxdal, D. S., Ferreira, A. A., and Scott, W. W. Estrogen inhibition of androgen-maintained prostatic secretion in the hypophysectomized dog. *J. Urol.* **86**:134, 1961.

6. Scott, W. W., and Schirmer, H. K. A. Hypophysectomy for disseminated prostatic cancer. In *On Cancer and Hormones*, University of Chicago Press, Chicago, 1962.
7. Scott, W. W. Growth and development of the human prostate. In *Biology of the Prostate and Related Tissues*, U.S.P.H. Monograph No. 12, p. 111, 1963.
8. Walton, K. N., Schirmer, H. K. A., and Scott, W. W. The effect of prolonged stimulation with pilocarpine upon secretory and metabolic activity of normal dog prostate gland. *Invest. Urol.* 1:23, 1963.
9. Walton, K. N., Schirmer, K. A., and Scott, W. W. Cholinesterase activity in the dog prostate gland. *Invest. Urol.* 1:307, 1964.
10. Kirchheim, D., Gyorkey, F., Brandes, D., and Scott, W. W. Histochemistry of the normal, hyperplastic, and neoplastic human prostate gland. *Invest. Urol.* 1:403, 1964.
11. Schirmer, K. A., Walton, K. N., and Scott, W. W. Prostatic epithelial cells: Their preparation and catalase activity. *Invest. Urol.* 1:301, 1964.
12. Tesar, C., and Scott, W. W. A search for inhibitors of prostate growth stimulators. *Invest. Urol.* 1:482, 1964.
13. Robson, M. C., and Scott, W. W. Effect of portal diversion of testicular blood on prostatic secretion in the dog. *Invest. Urol.* 1:92, 1964.
14. Bridge, R. W., and Scott, W. W. A new antiandrogen, SH-714, *Invest. Urol.* 2:99, 1964.
15. Brandes, D., Kirchheim, D., and Scott, W. W. Ultrastructure of the human prostate: Normal and neoplastic. *Lab. Invest.* 13:1541, 1964.
16. Campbell, E. W., Jr., and Scott, W. W. The effect of thyroxine and thiouracil on prostatic growth in the castrate male rat. *Invest. Urol.* 2:387, 1965.
17. Kirchheim, D., and Scott, W. W. The effect of castration and sex hormones upon aminopeptidase and phosphotases of the rat prostate. *Invest. Urol.* 2:393, 1965.
18. Scott, W. W., and Schirmer, H. K. A. A new oral progestational steroid effective in the treatment of prostatic cancer. *Trans. Am. Assoc. Genitourin. Surg.* 58:54, 1966.
19. Scott, W. W., and Wade, J. C. Medical treatment of benign nodular prostatic hyperplasia with cyproterone acetate. *J. Urol.* 101:81, 1969.

INTRODUCTION

In the castrate rat the androgen-induced growth in the ventral prostate gland is marked by two distinct characteristic processes. One component is the increase in the hypertrophic elements of the cell as measured by an increase in RNA and protein synthesis. These events occur very rapidly, and significant increases are noted within a few hours following initiation of hormone treatment. In contrast, the hyperplastic growth, which is marked by an increase in DNA synthesis and the subsequent cell division, is a late event following androgen treatment and occurs after a lag period of about 48 hr. These effects are typical of many mammalian systems which can be induced into growth by a variety of stimuli in that they have very characteristic and common phases. This has been described by Howard and Pelc[1] and popularized by Baserga[2] in a cell cycle which is depicted in Fig. 1. Following stimulation, a period is observed which is called the G_1 phase and is characterized by the rapid synthesis of RNA and proteins. The S phase, which marks the beginning of DNA synthesis, starts at 48 hr and is the time in which the cell duplicates the total DNA content of the cell.

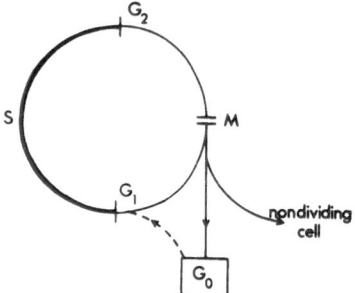

Fig. 1. Cell cycle as proposed by Howard and Pelc (from Baserga). M, mitosis, from prophase to telophase; G_1, interval between completion of mitosis and onset of DNA synthesis; S, period of DNA replication; G_2, interval between completion of DNA synthesis and mitosis; G_0, quiescent cells that can be stimulated to synthesize DNA and divide.

When this DNA synthesis ceases, a third period is observed which is termed the G_2 phase and is marked by a series of biochemical events that precedes the mitosis and cell division that ultimately produces the two daughter cells.

The present study was designed to determine when androgens are required in this type of cell cycle during prostatic growth. For example, is testosterone required to initiate the cell cycle but not required during the S period of DNA synthesis? This problem was approached by displacing the androgens from the prostatic nuclei by the application of cyproterone acetate, at specific time intervals in various growth phases. It is well established that the antiandrogen cyproterone acetate is capable of competing with testosterone and dihydrotestosterone in the prostatic nucleus[3-5]. The effects of displacing these androgens on a temporal scale are important because the current concepts of the mechanism of androgen action have visualized the interaction of the hormone with certain specific nuclear proteins and their subsequent release of genetic repression, which is expressed in the increase of RNA, DNA, and protein synthesis[6,7].

MATERIALS AND METHODS

Animals

Adult male albino rats of the Sprague–Dawley strain (250–350 g) were purchased from Huntingdon Farms. They were maintained on a diet of Purina Laboratory Chow and water *ad libitum* under a constant 12-hr light, 12-hr dark lighting schedule. Subcutaneous injections of testosterone propionate and cyproterone acetate dissolved in sesame oil were performed at the same time each day under conditions described in the text. Orchiectomy was performed via the scrotal route under ether anesthesia, and the animals were maintained for 5 days prior to therapy.

Cyproterone acetate was kindly provided by the Berlin Laboratories, New York, N.Y.

Incorporation of Radioactive Thymidine into DNA by Prostatic Minces in Vitro

Minced ventral prostate tissue (150 mg wet weight) was incubated at 37 C in 5 ml of medium containing 122 mM NaCl, 1.3 mM MgSO$_4$, 10 mM glucose, and 17.5 mM sodium phosphate, pH 7.4, with oxygen as the gas phase. The radioactive substrate was 0.048 mM of thymidine-methyl-H^3 (160 × 10^6 cpm/μmole). After a 60-min incubation with gentle shaking the reaction was stopped by the addition of 5 ml of cold 6% (w/v) trichloroacetic acid, (TCA), containing 0.1 mg of unlabeled thymidine per milliliter. The precipitate was centrifuged and washed three times with 6% TCA containing 0.1% thymidine (w/v) with 5 ml of 3:1 ethanol–ether (v/v) containing 1% potassium acetate. The final acid-insoluble precipitate was suspended in 2 ml of 1.6 N perchloric acid and heated for 20 min at 70 C. The extract was centrifuged at 40,000 × g for 5 min. The amount of isotope incorporated into the acid-soluble fraction was determined and correlated with the DNA (deoxyribose) content by the diphenylamine assay. The incorporation of thymidine into DNA was linear with time up to 90 min and with tissue weight.

Radioactivity was assayed with a Nuclear Chicago Unilux I liquid scintillation counter in 15 ml of a scintillation medium of the following composition: xylene–dioxane–absolute ethanol (1:1:1.1) containing 7.5% (w/v) naphthalene, 0.45% (w/v) 2,5-diphenyloxazole (Pilot Chemicals), and 0.0045% (w/v) 1,4-bis-(5-phenyloxazole-2-yl) benzene (Pilot Chemicals).

Preparation of Cell Nuclei

Prostatic cell nuclei were isolated by a modification of the procedure of Coffy et al[8]. Fresh ventral prostate tissue was placed in an iced vessel and minced thoroughly with scissors. A glass homogenizer equipped with a Teflon pestle was used to homogenize the mince at 2 C with 10 vol of 2.2 M sucrose containing 1 mM MgSO$_4$ and 5 mM β-mercaptoethanol. After filtration of the homogenate through silk cloth, the material was centrifuged for 1 hr at 50,000 × g at 2 C in a swinging-bucket rotor of a Beckman model L-2 ultracentrifuge. The cell nuclei, recovered in the pellet at the bottom of the tube, contained 58–72% of the total cellular DNA of the homogenate.

Prostatic Uptake of Testosterone-H^3

Fifty microcuries of testosterone-1,2-H^3 (specific activity 50 c/mmole, New England Nuclear Corp.) was dissolved in 0.5 ml of 0.9% NaCl and injected intraperitoneally 1 hr prior to sacrifice. The radioactivity was determined in the isolated nuclei. The disintegrations per minute are expressed per 100 μg of nuclear DNA. Preliminary experiments indicated that maximum uptake of label in the nucleus occurred at approximately 1 hr.

RESULTS

The postcastrate regression of the rat ventral prostate is accompanied by a rapid decline in the total RNA, DNA, and protein content of the gland. The loss in RNA and protein largely reflects the loss of cytoplasmic ribosomes and the shrinkage of the cytoplasm of the epithelial cells. The fall in the total amount of prostatic DNA after orchiectomy very probably reflects a decline in the total number of cells in the organ since there is no evidence for extensive occurrence of polyploidy or multinucleate epithelial cells in the prostate.

The system employed in these studies is a modification of the procedure of Tesar and Scott[9] and utilizes the restoration of ventral prostatic growth in the castrate rat by the administration of 0.2 mg per day of testosterone propionate for a period of 7 days. This treatment is capable of restoring the growth of the prostate and is denoted by the increase in the weight and the DNA, RNA, and protein content of the gland (Fig. 2). Simultaneous administration of cyproterone acetate (SH-714) was capable of blocking this restoration and clearly demonstrates its well-known antiandrogen effects[10]. This is in contrast to the synergistic effects observed when testosterone propionate and estradiol were given simultaneously, as was reported by Tesar and Scott.

In the present study attention was focused on the temporal events occurring during the initiation of DNA synthesis in the rat ventral prostate. In Fig. 3 it is apparent that the total DNA content of the rat ventral prostate is markedly decreased by castration. Exogenous testosterone propionate administration was begun on day 0 and continued daily for a period of 7 days. An initial lag period of 48 hr occurred before any significant increase was noted in the total DNA content of the gland; by 7 days the DNA content was restored to a normal value. However, if the rat was simultaneously treated with cyproterone acetate on each day, the accumulation of DNA was completely blocked.

DNA synthesis was measured by the incorporation of the thymidine precursor of DNA in an *in vitro* system. The rate of DNA synthesis was very low in the normal and castrate animals. When the castrate was given daily injections of testosterone, the 48-hr lag period was observed to be followed by a peak in DNA synthesis occurring at 3 days or 72 hr. DNA synthesis then subsided to normal levels even though the animals continued to receive daily injections of testosterone propionate. In the presence of

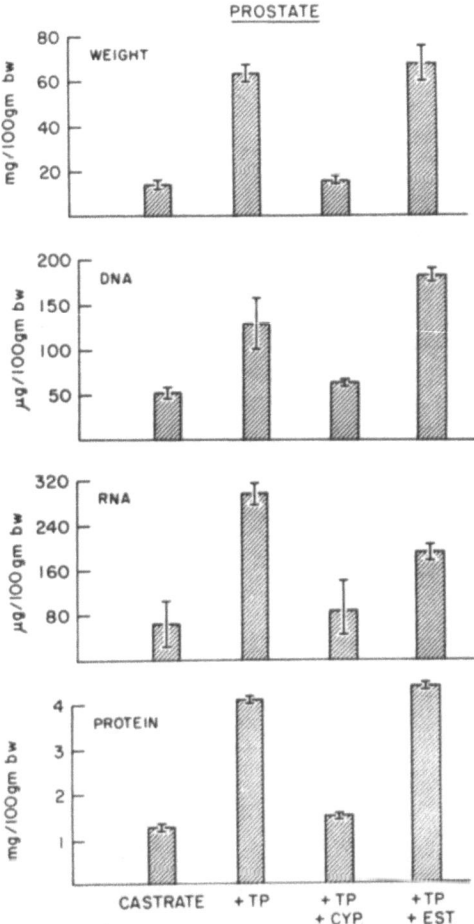

Fig. 2. The effects of 1 week of hormone treatment on the weight and DNA, RNA, and protein content of the castrate ventral prostate. TP, 0.2 mg of testosterone propionate per day; CYP, 6.0 mg of cyproterone acetate per day; EST, 2 mg of β-estradiol per day.

cyproterone acetate given *in vivo*, the pronounced increase in the rate of DNA synthesis at 3 days was completely inhibited.

Cyproterone acetate clearly blocks the DNA synthesis that is produced by androgen when the cyproterone is given in a thirtyfold excess over the amount of testosterone propionate. However, this inhibition could be completely overcome by injecting ten times the original dose of testosterone propionate (Fig. 4). This demonstrated that the cyproterone acetate was competing directly with testosterone to prevent the induction of DNA synthesis.

Several studies have indicated that cyproterone acetate is capable of blocking the uptake of labeled testosterone into the nucleus of prostatic cells[3-5]. This has been confirmed under the present experimental conditions. In the experiment summarized in Table 1, castrate animals were treated for 3 days with testosterone propionate. On the third day an intraperitoneal pulse of testosterone-H^3 was administered and the retention of the label was measured in the isolate nuclei.

It appears that cyproterone acetate was capable of inhibiting this uptake of labeled androgen. Fang and Liao[3] were able to demonstrate that this

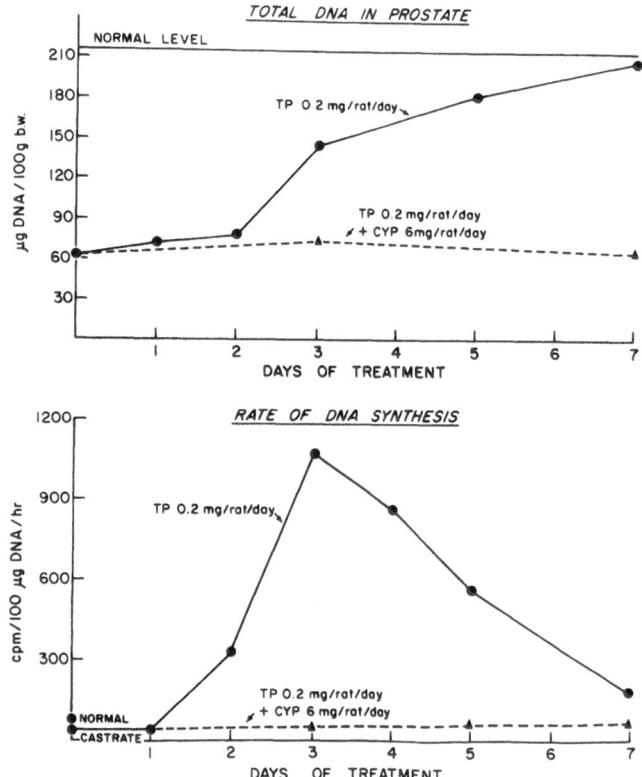

Fig. 3. The effects of testosterone propionate and cyproterone acetate on the accumulation of DNA in the ventral prostate gland and on the rate of DNA synthesis measured *in vitro* (see Materials and Methods).

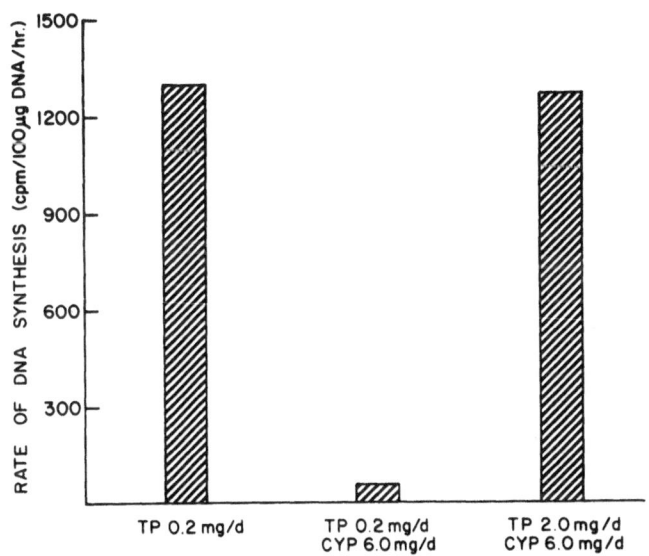

Fig. 4. The reversal of the cyproterone acetate inhibition of DNA synthesis by elevated doses of testosterone propionate.

Table 1. Effects of Cyproterone Acetate on the Retention of Androgens by Ventral Prostate Nuclei in Vivo

Treatment of castrates	Radioactive androgen associated with prostate nuclei	
	dpm/100 μg DNA	% inhibition
Testosterone	1985	
Testosterone and cyproterone	735	63

degree of inhibition essentially depleted the nucleus of the androgens which were associated with the specific nuclear protein receptors. The remaining label was associated with nonspecific binding in the nucleus.

The blockage of DNA synthesis and the inhibition of androgen uptake into the nucleus by cyproterone acetate permitted a study of the requirements of testosterone in the temporal events which precede DNA synthesis. As shown in Fig. 3, a 48-hr lag period ensued before the rate of DNA synthesis reached a peak at 72 hr. This permitted the application of cyproterone acetate at various intervals following the administration of testosterone propionate. In the experiment outlined in Fig. 5, all of the castrate animals received daily injections of testosterone propionate, and at the end of 72 hr the rate of DNA synthesis was measured by the incorporation of labeled thymidine into the DNA of the cell. If cyproterone

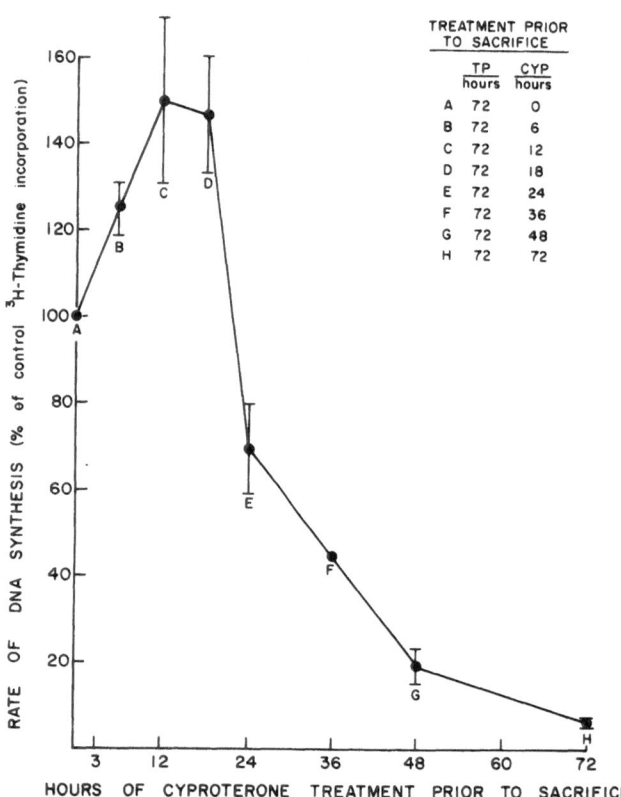

Fig. 5. The effects of treatment with cyproterone acetate for various time periods prior to sacrifice on DNA synthesis in the ventral prostate observed in castrates at 3 days following testosterone propionate injections. TP, 0.2 mg testosterone propionate per day for 3 days. CYP, 6.0 mg per day for various times as indicated.

acetate was given simultaneously with testosterone for the 72 hr, it completely blocked the DNA synthesis. However, if cyproterone acetate administration was delayed, a period was finally reached at which time cyptoterone acetate was completely ineffective in blocking DNA synthesis. This occurred at about 18–24 hr. At this time, cyproterone acetate did not block DNA synthesis; in fact, it produced significant stimulation. The cause of this stimulation is not known at present, but it cannot be explained by changes in pool size or changes in thymidine kinase activity. This was confirmed by using other precursors which are incorporated into DNA such as labeled formate or glycine.

It is concluded from the results shown in Fig. 5 and Fig. 3 that cyproterone acetate is capable of blocking DNA synthesis in the prostate only when given in the 48-hr period (G_1 phase) which precedes the initiation of DNA synthesis. In the experiment summarized in Table 2, an attempt was made to magnify this phenomenon by withholding testosterone treatment during the last 24 hr of the 72-hr period. In addition, during the last 24 hr cyproterone acetate was given at very high levels. This evidence clearly indicates that the cyproterone acetate which displaces the androgen is not capable of blocking DNA synthesis in the S period of cell cycle in prostatic tissue.

DISCUSSION

A 30:1 ratio of cyproterone acetate to testosterone propionate has been demonstrated to compete for most of the effective androgen-binding sites in the prostate and seminal vesicles[4]. In these studies a similiar ratio was sufficient to completely block the effects of testosterone propionate on the androgen-induced growth of the prostate in the castrate rat. The ability of cyproterone acetate to effectively compete for the androgen-binding sites in the prostate has been used here as a probe to study the requirements for androgens in various parts of the cell cycle of the prostate. Administration of exogenous testosterone propionate to the castrate rat is followed by a 48-hr lag period preceding the onset of DNA synthesis. This lag phase, termed the G_1 phase, is consistent with that observed in several mammalian systems induced into growth by a variety of stimuli. From this study it is apparent that cyproterone is capable of blocking DNA synthesis when given in the G_1 period but cannot block the synthesis of DNA in the S period. This might indicate that androgens are prerequisite for DNA synthesis but their presence is not really required during the synthesis S phase. This study is the first indication that a hormone does not have to be bound to a nuclear element at the time of the biosynthesis of DNA. Therefore, models employing the binding of the hormone to nuclear elements in the control of genome

Table 2. The Effect on DNA Synthesis of Withholding
Testosterone Treatment

Injection on days			DNA synthesis on day 3 (cpm/100 μg DNA)
1	2	3	
None	None	None	53
T	T	T	1738
T	T	None	1315
T	T	CYP	1765

expression are not within themselves sufficient to explain the control of DNA synthesis.

In addition, this study provides insight into the particular phase of the cell cycle which is blocked by cyproterone acetate therapy. This would appear to be pertinent information, since the hyperplastic phase of prostatic growth accounts for many of the pathological conditions occurring in the human prostate and cyproterone acetate is providing a new means of therapy in the control of those diseases([11,12]).

REFERENCES

1. Howard, A., and Pelc, S. R. Nuclear incorporation of P-32 as demonstrated by autoradiographs. *Exptl. Cell Res.* 2:178, 1951.
2. Baserga, R. *Biochemistry of Cell Division,* Charles C. Thomas, Publisher, Springfield, Ill., pp. 3–5, 1969
3. Fang, S., and Liao, S. Antagonistic action of anti-androgens on the formation of a specific dihydrotestosterone receptor protein complex in rat ventral prostate. *Molec. Pharmacol.* 5:420, 1969.
4. Stein, J. M., and Eisenfeld, A. J. Androgen accumulation and binding to macromolecules in seminal vesicles: Inhibition by cyproterone acetate. *Science* 166:233, 1969.
5. Fang, S., Anderson, K. M., and Liao, S. Receptor proteins for androgens. *J. Biol. Chem.* 244: 6584, 1969.
6. Liao, S., Barton, R. W., and Lin, A. H. Differential synthesis of ribonucleic acid in prostatic nuclei: Evidence for selective gene transcription induced by androgens. *Proc. Natl. Acad. Sci.* 55:1593, 1966.
7. Liao, S., and Fang, S. Receptor-proteins for androgens and the mode of action of androgens on gene transcription in ventral prostate. *Vitamins and Hormones* 27:17, 1970.
8. Coffey, D. S., Shimazaki, J., and Williams-Ashman, H. G. Polymerization of deoxyribonucleotides in relation to androgen-induced prostatic growth. *Arch. Biochem. Biophys.* 24:184, 1968.
9. Tesar, C., and Scott, W. W. A search for inhibitors of prostatic growth stimulators. *Invest. Urol.* 1:482, 1964.
10. Bridge, R. W., and Scott, W. W. A new antiandrogen, SH-714. *Invest. Urol.* 2:99, 1964.
11. Scott, W. W., and Schirmer, H. K. A. A new oral progestational steroid effective in treating prostatic cancer. *Trans. Am. Assoc. Genitourin. Surg.* 58:54, 1966.
12. Scott, W. W., and Wade, J. C. Medical treatment of benign nodular prostatic hyperplasia with cyproterone acetate. *J. Urol.* 101:81, 1969.

Reflections on the Etiology of Benign Prostatic Hypertrophy

John T. Grayhack*

Biased written speculation is usually avoided by most of us, scientists, pseudoscientists, or what have you, since the risk of error and ridicule outweigh the potential personal rewards and public good. However, the man we are honoring by this effort, Professor W. W. Scott, has characterized his relationship with us by an attitude of tolerance toward our indiscretions and encouragement for our sincere individual efforts without placing a value judgment on them. His attitude and the security of our friendships encourage me to present a brief, selective summary of observations concerning benign prostatic hypertrophy and prostatic growth in man and animals and to attempt to relate them to each other.

THE PROBLEM

So-called benign prostatic hypertrophy is a fibromuscular glandular hyperplasia of the prostate that occurs in the prostate of the human male as he ages. Although other aging animals such as the dog exhibit a diffuse hyperplasia of the prostate, the characteristic nodular hypertrophy of man is unique. Histological studies indicate that benign prostatic hypertrophy usually begins in the inner or suburethral prostatic glands. Either stromal or epithelial changes may initiate or predominate in this process[1,2]. Although atrophic changes in the peripheral prostatic glands may accompany

*Department of Urology, Northwestern University Medical School, Evanston, Illinois.

the proliferation of the periurethral elements, weight[3] and volume[4] studies indicate that the overall size of the prostate of man increases with aging. Histological evidence of benign prostatic hypertrophy is present in most, not all, men over 60 years of age[5].

When evaluated in terms of our usual understanding of factors controlling accessory sex gland growth, this increase in size of the prostate with aging seems paradoxical. The physiological dependence of male accessory sex glands on testicular function for growth and maintenance is recognized and readily demonstrable. The bulk of experimental evidence suggests that testicular control of accessory sex gland growth is mediated by androgen secretion. The probability that the nature and quantity of this secretion varies with age is great. Studies of plasma levels of androsterone and dehydroepiandrosterone indicate a gradual decrease with aging starting in the mid-twenties[6]. The studies of urinary excretion of steroids and more impressively biological androgens reveal a similar trend[7,8]. Determinations of plasma and urinary testosterone have not indicated a uniform trend, although testosterone secretory and excretory rates seem to be depressed in the older male[9,10]. A variety of studies suggest that the capacity of the testis to synthesize androgens declines as a function of age[11].

This combination of increasing accessory sex gland growth with evidence of decreasing testicular function raises two primary questions with regard to prostatic growth noted in the aging human male: (a) is it a stimulated growth? and (b) is it under continuing control or does it achieve independent growth status?

IS PROSTATIC GROWTH OF THE AGING MALE STIMULATED?

Although patients with some degree of hypogonadism, such as those with Klinefelter's syndrome, have been observed to develop benign prostatic hypertrophy[12], this growth has not been reported in a male deprived of his testes in youth[1]. The number of observations documenting this statement is limited, but its validity is reinforced by the absence of any reported exception. The testes, therefore, seem necessary for the continuing prostatic growth of the aging male. The role they play might vary from one of direct stimulation to simply maintenance of sufficient metabolic activity to allow pathological changes to be induced or occur.

Recently, evidence has accumulated that the active stimulant to epithelial cell growth in the prostate may be dihydrotestosterone (17β-hydroxy-5α-androstan-3-one) rather than testosterone itself[13]. Testosterone is thought to be converted to dihydrotestosterone in the cytosol. The dihydrotestosterone then combines with a specific macromolecule and enters the nucleus (Fig. 1), where it may well play a role in the stimulation of

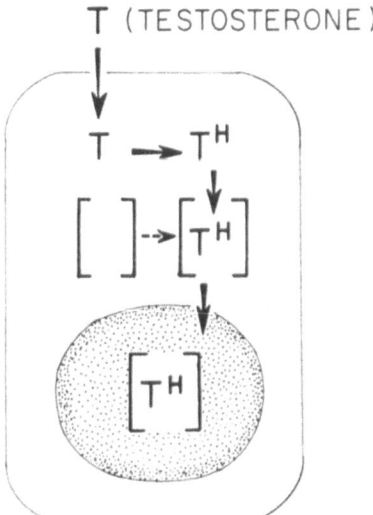

T (TESTOSTERONE)

Fig. 1. Schematic representation of probable relationship of testosterone and dihydrotestosterone in prostatic epithelial cell. Testosterone (T) is converted to dihydrotestosterone (T^H) in the cytosol. The dihydrotestosterone is bound by a specific macromolecule. The bound dihydrotestosterone enters the nucleus where it presumably catalyzes protein synthesis. Testosterone probably also enters the nucleus and participates in metabolic changes.

protein synthesis[14-16]. Knowledge of this new concept led Sitteri and Wilson[17] to determine the dihydrotestosterone and testosterone concentration of epithelial cells of the prostate of men of varying ages. Benign prostatic hypertrophy and normal prostatic tissue were also compared. Surprisingly, the dihydrotestosterone concentration was higher in old men than in young men; benign prostatic hypertrophic tissue had five times as much dihydrotestosterone as normal tissue. In addition, the periurethral prostatic tissue was found to have a disproportionately high dihydrotestosterone content prior to the development of recognized hypertrophy. These observations lend considerable support to a significant direct stimulatory role of the testes and androgens in the genesis of benign prostatic hypertrophy.

IS BENIGN PROSTATIC HYPERTROPHY UNDER CONTINUING ENDROCINE CONTROL?

The possibility that endocrine stimulation might be essential to the initial but not to the continuing growth of benign prostatic hypertrophy raises a legitimate question that has important therapeutic consequences. Previous therapeutic endeavors shed some insight on the problem. Castration has been performed for benign prostatic hypertrophy sporadically since the end of the last century. White[18] reported a decrease in prostate size in 65 of 102 patients with an unconfirmed diagnosis of benign prostatic hypertrophy. Huggins and Stevens[19] noted a similar change in one of three patients subjected to castration. Deming[20] observed no change in prostatic size in a 1-month period following castration and referred to several reports of similar failure of response to this procedure. Huggins and Stevens reported a decrease in acinar size in two of three patients 86 and 91 days after castration. Recently, Wendel *et al.*[21] have studied the histological characteristics of benign prostatic hypertrophy at autopsy in three groups of patients: (a) patients with carcinoma of the prostate subjected to orchiectomy with or without concomitant estrogen administration for at least 3 months prior to death, (b) patients with untreated carcinoma in various stages discovered at autopsy, and (3) a series of selected matching patients to serve as controls. The configuration of the acini, the degree of epithelial infolding, and the cellular characteristics of the groups were evaluated. The control and untreated carcinomas of the prostate groups were comparable with regard to each parameter; the patients subjected to orchiectomy and estrogen showed uniform evidence of decreased epithelial stimulation of the portion of the prostate gland involved in benign hypertrophy.

In addition to the observations with regard to the effect of castration on benign prostatic hypertrophy, the literature is replete with reports of therapeutic effects of varying steroids on this lesion. Estrogens, androgens, estrogen–androgen mixtures, and progestational agents have all been reported to affect the size of the prostate or the degree of bladder neck obstruction[22–25]. Most of these observations have not been rigidly controlled. They amount to unsubstantiated claims, many of which have been unconfirmed on repeated subsequent trials. However, the studies of Scott and Wade[24] with cyproterone acetate and Geller[27] with hydroxyprogesterone caproate are of special interest. Both lack totally adequate control observations, but the studies carried out include evaluation of prostatic size and histology, as well as some assessment of the degree of bladder neck obstruction. The results of their observations indicate a responsiveness of benign prostatic hypertrophy to steroid administration.

The evidence suggesting that benign prostatic hypertrophy is under continuing endocrine stimulation is fragmented and usually derived from a clinical study that has necessitated a compromise with an ideal group of observations. Nevertheless, the combination of the findings in castrated males and those subjected to administration of various steroids suggests that benign prostatic hypertrophy is under continuing hormonal stimulation. This leads to a final question, namely, if benign prostatic hypertrophy is initiated and maintained by endocrine secretion, what are the source and nature of these secretions?

BPH—INITIATED AND MAINTAINED BY WHAT?

The assumptions that the male accessory sex organs are stimulated only by androgens and that chemical or biological determinations of androgens in blood or urine assess accurately and totally accessory sex gland–stimulating substances warrant careful scrutiny and question. A number of nonandrogenic hormones have been shown to be capable of stimulating the prostate of animals. Histological study demonstrates a marked increase in fibromuscular tissue of the prostate of monkeys and an epithelial stimulation of the prostate of dogs and rodents following estrogen administration[28–31]. Estrone and estradiol administered with testosterone to castrate rats have been shown to increase weight of the dorsal lateral and lateral lobes of the prostate[32,33]. The citric acid content and concentration of the lateral lobes of the rat prostate have been markedly increased by the combined administration of estradiol and testosterone. The administration of somatotrophin and prolactin in conjunction with testosterone has resulted in an increased weight of the rat prostate[34,35]. The increase in weight noted following prolactin is again most pronounced in the lateral lobe and is associated with an increase in citric acid content and concentration. These selected examples demonstrate the assumption that accessory sex gland stimulation in a variety of male animals is confined to the usual group of steroids reconized as androgenic is unwarranted. The relationship of the observations in animals to accessory sex gland growth in man remains uncertain.

The problems inherent in attempting to assess the absolute amounts of a given steroid secreted and reaching an accessory sex gland in an active form by chemical determination of the steroid or its metabolites in blood or urine are recognized by those who carry out or seek to evaluate these studies. Determinations of biological activity in the urine may reflect a change in the secretory rate of androgens, a variation in the metabolic conversion of the secreted androgen, or a variety of factors affecting the assay itself. Neither chemical nor biological tests seem likely to represent absolute secretory or systemic androgen levels accurately. The hope for a stable relation between determined and actual values does not seem unrealistic. Nevertheless, the possibility that attempts to quantitate the male accessory sex gland–stimulating substances present represent an incomplete or misdirected effort cannot be dismissed. For these reasons, we attempted to assess the hormonal stimuli to accessory sex gland growth in man by utilizing various gravimetric and biochemical indicators employed to assay these stimuli in animals. Wet and dry weights as well as fructose concentration of the fluid were determined in seminal vesicles obtained at autopsy from 196 men[36]. A progressive decline in the fructose concentration was associated with maintenance of wet and dry vesicle weight. The weight maintenance of this accessory sex organ suggests continuing accessory sex gland stimulation; the failure to maintain the fructose level of the vesicle fluid suggests that the continuing stimulation is not due primarily to an androgen. A similar conclusion was suggested by the observations of citric acid, acid phosphatase, and lactic dehydrogenase concentration of the expressed prostatic fluid of men of varying ages. The citric acid concentration increased unexpectedly to its highest levels in the 40- to 59-year-old age group; the levels in the 59 and over and 20–40 age groups were essentially comparable. On the other hand, both acid phosphatase and lactic dehydrogenase levels declined progressively with age[37].

We have been encouraged by these observations to attempt to demonstrate the presence of accessory sex gland–stimulating substances in the aging male which differ from recognized androgenic steroids. The possibility that estrogenic substances may be the stimulus that act synergistically with androgen and result in continuing prostatic growth has been postulated repeatedly and warrants major consideration[1]. The less prominent possibility of a nonsteroidal stimulus to prostatic growth has dominated our efforts. Our group has attempted to obtain evidence for the presence of non-androgenic accessory sex gland–stimulating substances in the aging male in three ways:

1. An attempt was made to identify an extractable growth hormone-lactogen-like protein in the testis by immunological studies of ovine[38] and human testicular extracts[39,40]. Double gel diffusion studies suggested an antigenic similarity between testicular extracts and growth hormone. Biological tests yielded variable results. Seminal vesicle weight and the width of the tibial epiphyseal plate were increased in hypophysectomized rats following the administration of the testicular extract. Lactation was produced in the pseudopregnant rabbit in only one of several attempts. Crop sac assays in pigeons yielded no evidence of activity. The inconstancy of biological activity and the discovery of a reactive antigen in extracts of stomach and ovary (but not liver or kidney) lessened our enthusiasm for the extraction procedures. At the present time, perfusion studies of the testis are being attempted in an effort to improve the quality and quantity of testicular protein available for study.

2. A crude filtrate of male urine was obtained by passing it through a millipore filter with 10,000 mw pore size[41]. The retention of steroids by this technique seemed improbable. The diaflo concentrate was then lyophilized. The resulting material was suspended in saline and injected subcutaneously daily for 14 days in rats that had been hypophysectomized and orchiectomized for over 3 weeks. Testosterone propionate in oil was administered subcutaneously in 1 mg amounts every other day. Five separate preparations of urine were tested in three separate experiments. The results

of the last of these experiments in which a nonspecific protein, egg albumin, was utilized as an additional control are presented in Table 1. As in the data presented, the mean weight of the lateral lobe of the prostate exceeded that of the control in each experiment. The changes in citric acid content of this lobe add suggestive evidence of metabolic stimulation. Urine from women and castrate males did not increase weight of the lateral or other lobes of the prostate of a small group of hypophysectomized castrate animals injected with testosterone propionate. In the absence of androgen, no response to male urine extract was noted.

    3.   An end-organ androgenic antagonist, 6α-bromo-17β-hydroxy-17α-methyl-4-oxa-5α-androstan-3-one (RO7-2340)([42]), was administered to intact male rats with the hope that its administration would result in endogenous stimulation of testicular secretion([43]). It was postulated that this would result in an excess secretion with an uninhibited end-organ effect of nonandrogenic hormones and that this might manifest itself by a differing growth or regression rate of the various lobes of the prostate in response to the antiandrogen. In pilot experiments the suppressive effect of RO7-2340 on the weight of the ventral, lateral, and dorsal prostate of young adult males was similar; in older animals, retired breeders, the weight of the lateral lobes seemed to be proportionately less depressed than the ventral and dorsal lobes of the prostate. Currently this problem is being evaluated further. Table 2 presents the weight of the prostatic lobes in a group of retired breeders given 6 mg of RO7-2340 for 14 days and then sacrificed 1 day after the final injection. As the data presented in Table 2 illustrate, there is a disproportionate maintenance of the weight response of the lateral lobe of the prostate. Administration of testosterone propionate 0.5 mg every other day and RO7-2340 6 mg daily to castrate rats produced no disproportionate weight response of the lateral lobes, suggesting that the results

Table 1. Results of Experiment to Determine Effect of Human Urine Filtrate and Egg Albumin on Castrate Rat Prostate[a,c]

Rat	No.	Final body weight (g)	Prostate weight[b] mg			Citric acid[b] (μg/organ)	Fructose[b] (μg/organ)
			Ventral	Lateral	Dorsal		
Control	16	152	283 ± 34	99 ± 13	92 ± 16	14 ± 6	73 ± 22
Human urine							
filtrate	10	154	291 ± 44	111 ± 16	103 ± 17	23 ± 10	79 ± 24
Albumin	13	147	313 ± 44	102 ± 10	104 ± 14	13 ± 4	71 ± 16

[a] Body weight, weight of ventral, dorsal, and lateral lobe of prostate, and citric acid and fructose content of lateral lobe of prostate of hypophysectomized castrate Sprague–Dawley rats injected with 1 mg testosterone propionate in oil every other day for 14 days. In addition, 13 rats received 10 mg chicken egg albumin and ten received 10 mg protein obtained by passing human male urine through 10,000 mw millipore filter subcutaneously daily.
[b] $\pm$ SD.
[c] Since submission for publication attempts to reproduce these data have yielded variable results.

Table 2. Results of Experiment to Determine Effect of RO7-2340 on Castrate Rat Prostate[a]

Rat	No.	Steroid	Prostate weight[b] (g)			Relative change prostate weight[b]		
			Ventral	Lateral	Dorsal	Ventral/lateral	Ventral/dorsal	Dorsal/lateral
Normal	11	—	782±168	224±45	139±31	3.52±0.60	5.70±0.91	0.620±0.07
Normal	11	6 mg RO7-2340	663±192	228±59	123±33	3.02±0.89	5.65±1.96	0.564±0.17
Castrate	8	0.5 mg TP	991±113	323±60	160±13	3.16±0.74	6.21±0.59	0.504±0.08
Castrate	6	0.5 mg TP 6 mg RO7-2340	778±156	213±35	144±16	3.67±0.51	5.16±1.45	0.693±0.126
Castrate	5	0.5 mg TP 12 mg RO7-2340	675±181	203±70	143±14	3.52±1.028	4.83±1.70	0.783±0.29

[a] Summary of final prostate weights and ratio of weight changes of lobes of prostate of retired breeder Sprague–Dawley rats with intact testes given 6 mg 6α-bromo-17β-hydroxy-17α-methyl-4-oxa-5α-androstan-3-one (RO7-2340) 6 mg in oil daily for 14 days with autopsy 1 day following final injection. Similar observations in rats orchiectomized 26 days before initiating injection of testosterone propionate (T.P) 0.5 mg every other day for 14 days; rats receiving RO7-2340 daily in addition are indicated (Johnson, B., et al.: Unpublished data)[43].

[b] ±SD.

observed in the intact male animal were not the result of a synergism between these steroids with regard to the lateral lobe.

Unusual observations with regard to prostatic growth seem to be related primarily to an effect on the lateral lobe of the prostate of the rat. The inadvisability of attempting to transpose observations from one species to another are readily apparent, especially when the observations seem to be isolated to a portion of the accessory sexual apparatus. However, we are encouraged to emphasize these unusual responses by the suggestion of Price[44] that the lateral lobe of the rodent prostate is probably homologous to that portion of the prostate that we recognize as the usual site of benign prostatic hypertrophy and by the recognition that benign prostatic hypertrophy itself is a paradoxical alteration in a limited portion of the prostate.

Evidence presently available would suggest that the answer to the question "BPH—initiated and maintained by what?" should probably emphasize accessory sex gland–stimulating substances other than androgens. The evidence in animals supports the possibility of stimulation by nonandrogenic steroids and protein hormones. Each time evidence has been sought for an accessory sex gland–stimulating substance in addition to the usually recognized androgenic steroids in man, the observations have tended to support rather than refute this concept.

Currently our working hypothesis is that benign prostatic hypertrophy is initiated and maintained by endocrine stimulation. The nature of the endocrine stimulation seems likely to be a complex one in which androgen and another endocrine substance interact. Testosterone or a similar androgenic steroid secreted by the testis seems unquestionably to be necessary for the growth of the prostate of the aging male. However, a nonandrogenic substance that stimulates the conversion to or the retention of dihydrotestosterone by the periurethral prostatic cell seems likely to be the critical stimulant to the observed growth.

SUMMARY

Review of the evidence that suggests that benign prostatic hypertrophy is stimulated by and under continuing control of endocrine secretions reveals substantial support for both these concepts. Although the identity of these hormones as well as the mechanism of their action is uncertain, the concept that a nonandrogenic hormone plays a critical role in the prostatic growth pattern associated with aging warrants serious consideration. If the suggestion that benign prostatic hypertrophy is a stimulated and controlled growth is correct, the probability that the pathological process will be amenable to preventive and possibly to therapeutic measures utilizing information gained from continuing studies of hormone–prostate interrelationship seems great.

REFERENCES

1. Mostofi, F. K., and Thompson, R. V. Benign hyperplasia of the prostate gland. In Campbell, M. E. (ed.), *Urology,* 2nd ed., W. B. Saunders Company, Philadelphia, p. 1101, 1963.
2. Franks, L. M. Benign nodular hyperplasia of the prostate. A review. *Ann. Roy. Coll. Surg.* **14:** 92, 1954.
3. Teem, M. The relation of the interstitial cells of the testes to prostatic hypertrophy. *J. Urol.* **34:**692, 1935.
4. Swyer, G. I. M. Post-natal growth changes in the human prostate. *J. Anat.* **78:**130, 1944.
5. Moore, R. A. Benign hypertrophy of the prostate. A morphological study. *J. Urol.* **50:**680, 1943,
6. Migeon, C. J., Kelly, A. R., Lawrence, B., and Shephard, T. H. Dehydroepiandrosterone and androsterone levels in human plasma. Effect of age and sex: Day to day and diurnal variations. *J. Clin. Endocrinol.* **17:**1051, 1957.
7. Pincus, G. Aging and urinary steroid excretion. In Engle., E. J., and Pincus, G. (eds.), *Hormones and the Aging Process,* Academic Press, New York, 1955.
8. Pincus, G., Dorfman, I., Romanoff, L. P., Rubin, B. L., Bloch, E., Carlo, J., and Freehman, H. Steroid metabolism in aging men and women. *Recent Prog. Hormone Res.* **11:**307, 1955.
9. Vermeulen, A. *Androgens in Normal and Pathological Conditions,* Excerpta Medica Foundation, New York, 1966.
10. Morer-Forgas, F., and Nowakowski, H. Die Testosteronausscheidung im Harn bei männlichen Individuen. *Acta Endocrinol.* **49:**443, 1965.
11. Eik-Nes, K. B. Synthesis and secretion of androstanedione and testosterone. In Eik-Nes, K. B. (ed.), *The Androgens of the Testis,* Marcel Dekker, Inc., New York, 1970, p. 39.
12. Miller, H. C., and McDonald, P. F. Klinefelter's syndrome and benign prostatic hypertrophy. *J.A.M.A.* **186:**215, 1963.
13. Williams-Ashman, H. G. Biochemistry of testicular androgen action. In Eik-Nes, K. B. (ed.), *The Androgens of the Testis,* Marcel Dekker, Inc., New York, 1970, p. 121.
14. Mainwaring, W. I. P. A soluble androgen receptor in the cytoplasm of rat prostate. *J. Endocrinol.* **45:**531, 1969.
15. Fang, S., Anderson, K. M., and Liao, S. Receptor proteins for androgens. *J. Biol. Chem.* **244:**6584, 1969.
16. Liao, S., and Fang, S. Receptor proteins for androgens and the mode of action of androgens on gene transcription in ventral prostate. *Vitamins and Hormones* **27:**18, 1969.
17. Sitteri, P. K., and Wilson, J. D. The formation and content of dihydrotestosterone in hypertrophic prostate of man. *J. Clin. Invest.* **49:**1737, 1970.
18. White, W. The results of double castration in hypertrophy of the prostate. *Ann. Surg.* **22:**1, 1895.
19. Huggins, C., and Stevens, R. H. The effect of castration on benign hypertrophy of the prostate in man. *J. Urol.* **43:**705, 1940.
20. Deming, C. L., Jenkins, R. H., and Van Wagner, G. Some endocrinological relationships of prostatic hypertrophy. *J. Urol.* **33:**388, 1935.
21. Wendel, E., Putong, P., Brannon, G., and Grayhack, J. T. The effect of orchiectomy and estrogens on benign prostatic hyperplasia. Submitted for publication.
22. Kahle, P. S., and Maltry, E. Treatment of hyperplasia of the prostate with diethylstilbestrol dipropionate. *New Orleans Med. Surg. J.* **93:**121, 1941.
23. Pierson, E. L. A study of the effect of stilbestrol therapy on the size of the benign hypertrophied prostate gland. *J. Med.* **55:**73, 1946.

24. Walther, H. W. E., and Willoughby, R. M. Hormonal treatment of benign prostatic hyperplasia. *J. Urol.* **40**:135, 1938.
25. Kaufman, J. J., and Goodwin, W. E. Hormonal management of the benign obstructing prostate: Use of combined androgenic–estrogen therapy. *J. Urol.* **81**:165, 1959.
26. Scott, W. W., and Wade, J. C. Medical treatment of benign nodular prostatic hyperplasia with cyproterone acetate. *J. Urol.* **101**:81, 1969.
27. Geller, J., Angrist, A., Nakao, K., and Newman, H. Therapy with progestational agents in advanced benign prostatic hypertrophy. *J.A.M.A.* **210**:1421, 1969.
28. Von Wagenen, G. The effects of oestrone on the urogenital tract of the male monkey. *Anat. Rev.* **63**:387, 1945.
29. Berg, O. A. Effect of stilbestrol on prostate in normal puppies and adult dog. *Acta Endocrinol.* **27**:165, 1958.
30. Thorburg, J. V. On the influence of oestrogenic hormones on the male accessory genital system. *Acta Endocrinol. Suppl.*, p. 1, 1948.
31. Kovenchevsky, V., and Dennison, M. The effect of oestrone on normal and castrated male rats. *Biochem. J.* **28**:1474, 1934.
32. Grayhack, J. T., and Kretchmer, L. Response of the rat prostate to estrogen pellet implantation. *Invest. Urol.* **1**:121, 1963.
33. Grayhack, J. T. Effect of testosterone–estradiol administration on cirtic acid and fructose content of the rat prostate. *Endocrinology* **77**:1068, 1965.
34. Grayhack, J. T. Pituitary factors influencing growth of the prostate. In *Biology of Prostate and Related Tissues,* National Cancer Institute Monograph No. 12, p. 189, 1963.
35. Grayhack, J. T., and Lebowitz, J. M. Effect of prolactin on citric acid of lateral lobe of prostate of Sprague–Dawley rat. *Invest. Urol.* **5**:87, 1967.
36. Grayhack, J. T. Changes with aging in human seminal vesicle fluid fructose concentration and seminal vesicle weight. *J. Urol.* **86**:142, 1961.
37. Grayhack, J. T., and Kropp, K. A. Changes with aging in prostatic fluid citric acid, acid phosphatase, and lactic dehydrogenase concentration in man *J. Urol.* **93**:258, 1965.
38. Kaplan, G. W., Barrett, R. J., and Grayhack, J. T. Extraction of a substance with prolactin-like and growth hormone–like properties from ovine testes: Preliminary communication. *J. Urol.* **97**:494, 1967.
39. Barrett, R. J., Kaplan, G. W., Dahl, D., and Belman, A. B. Testicular proteins (TP) immunologically related to pituitary growth hormone. Proc. Third Internat. Congr. Endocrinol., p. 22, 1968 (July) (Excerpta Medica 157).
40. Barrett, R. J., Belman, A. B., Dahl, D., and Kaplan, G. W. Unpublished observations.
41. Wendel, E., and Grayhack, J. T. Unpublished observations.
42. Boris, A., and Uskokovic, M.: A new antinadrogen, 6α-bromo-17β-hydroxy-17α-methyl-4-oxa-5α-androstan-3-one. *Experientia* **26**:9, 1970.
43. Johnson, B., and Grayhack, J. T. Unpublished observations.
44. Price, D. Comparative aspects of development and structure in the prostate. In *Biology of Prostate and Related Tissues,* National Cancer Institute Monograph No. 12, p. 1, 1963.

Vesical Suspension in the Management of Obstructive Disease of the Bladder

J. N. DeKlerk*

Urologists have always accepted the truism that vesical outflow obstruction should be corrected whenever possible. Until comparatively recently, the efforts of all urological surgeons were directed toward relieving the commonly recognized forms of outflow obstructions, for example, bladder neck contracture or prostatic hyperplasia, but during the last decade a newer dimension has obtruded itself upon the scene.

Following the original work by Bradford Young and his colleagues[1-10] demonstrating that, in the female, obstructive disease of the bladder is a definite clinical entity, the fact slowly began to emerge that although numerous female patients were presenting with signs and symptoms compatible with obstructive disease of the bladder and its sequelae, in a very high percentage of cases no overt rigid obstructive lesion could be demonstrated in the bladder outflow.

Following upon the work of Paquin[12], numerous other investigators[13-15] were able to demonstrate that by using newer parameters of vesical function based upon flowmetric and hydrodynamic factors related to the flow of urine from the bladder through the urethra it was possible to postulate the presence of an anatomically nonrigid, nonovert, obstructive bladder malfunction.

It became clear that voiding efficiency is to a large extent qualified by urethral resistance, urethral tone, fluid turbulence, character of the urinary flow (whether centripetal or centrifugal), and the jet effect, and that this

*Department of Urology, Faculty of Medicine, University of Stellenbosch and the Karl Bremer Hospital, Bellville, South Africa.

multiplicity of hydrodynamic factors coupled with the efficacy of the detrusor function equally well determine whether or not the patient empties her or his bladder efficiently. It also became clear that for purposes of correct evaluation the *de facto* vesicourethral lumen should be regarded as one entity and that any alteration in the summated lines of hydrodynamic force governing the direction of urine flow from the bladder through the urethra can result in an altered efficiency of micturition.

This diminished vesical efficiency is as important a factor in the development of bladder pathology as any form of overt obstruction may be.

COMPARATIVE ANATOMICAL CONSIDERATIONS

In the quadruped mammal, the bladder is a largely abdominal organ which with increased filling is mainly supported by the rectus abdominis muscle and the other abdominal muscles. During the act of micturition, any elevation in abdominal pressure is in a dorsoventral direction, and there is no tendency for the bladder to be pushed caudally. The pelvic musculature plays a minimal supportive role and specifically provides no support to the bladder itself. In the human mammal, the situation is not greatly changed until the child commences to walk and assumes the erect position. From this stage onward, the bladder tends to become a pelvic organ rather than an abdominal one, and on distention the main support must now be provided by the pelvic floor as there are no other supportive ligaments or fascial layers capable of fulfilling this role. The vesical fascia and covering peritoneum play but a very minor role in this process. In the human male, the bladder depends chiefly for its stability on its attachment to the pubis via the pubovesical and puboprostatic ligaments; in the female, stablity depends on attachment via the pubocervical and/or pubovesical ligaments. In both the male and the female, the base of the bladder depends for its support almost entirely on the levator ani muscle and its fascia, and, as is anatomically well known, this muscle has numerous hiatuses, particularly in the female, which lend themselves readily to divarication and concomitant loss of pelvic support. In the erect position, the tendency is for the bladder to fall backward from its attachment at the pubovesical ligament, with a resultant angulation of the bladder cavity on the urethral lumen at the bladder neck. During the act of micturition in the erect or sitting position, this tendency is further aggravated by the downward displacement of the bladder relative to the bladder neck by increased intra-abdominal pressure.

It is also apparent that any condition tending to diminish the supportive role of the pelvic floor, such as, for example, pregnancy, poor muscular development, age, or iatrogenic factors including total hysterectomy and/or abdominoperineal resection, will greatly aggravate this situation.

Hutch[16] and numerous other workers[17-19] have clearly shown that in the initial stages of the act of normal micturition an important factor is the elimination of the dorsal urethrovesical angle. (This is of course unnecessary in the quadruped, where this dorsal urethrovesical angle does not exist.) It is clear from what has been discussed above that this essential preliminary factor in the act of micturition may become increasingly deficient if the factors responsible for preventing posteroinferior displacement of the bladder upon the bladder neck are absent or inefficient.

My feelings on the subject can best be summarized as follows: It is my opinion that the human bladder is at best a somewhat poor adaptation of the quadruped bladder. It is peculiarly inefficiently supported to take the strain of vesical filling and abdominal pressure downward. This lack of support, with its consequent posterior and downward displacement of the bladder relative to the fixed urethra and bladder neck, is basically always present in the erect human. It is, however, often further aggravated or accentuated by several additional factors. Under normal circumstances, for example, during the act of micturition, there may be a concomitant relaxation of the pelvic diaphragm, and therefore instead of the strong supporting action which would normally be required to combat the depressing effect of intraabdominal pressure on the bladder and its relation to the urethrovesical angle, the reverse now applies, and there is a tendency to counteract the normal decrease in the urethrovesical angle associated with the initiation of micturition.

Any condition which would normally affect the normal tone of the pelvic musculature could produce a similar set of circumstances, e.g., pregnancy and hyperprogesteronism. Iatrogenically, the same situation could be produced postoperatively after total hysterectomy or after abdominoperineal resection.

Lastly, we must not lose sight of the fact that this deficient support may be developmental in origin. Anatomically, it is possible to demonstrate considerable variation in the size and strength of the pelvic muscular diaphragm. A poorly developed pelvic floor is often associated with visceroptosis and lordosis; however, it is possible to demonstrate very severe posterior displacement of the base of the bladder with all the vesical features similar to early cystocele in a young prepubertal child in whom there is no possibility of an associated hormonal or other factor being present. This developmental abnormality may occur in both sexes equally.

CLINICAL FEATURES

Resultant upon this vesical malfunction, the patient may present in a host of different ways, varying to some extent according to age or sex but basically always with infection secondary to a deficient outflow. In a child, a common presenting symptom is urinary tract infection with or without a preceding history of enuresis. In such children, apart from the florid case presenting with obvious pyelographic evidence of upper urinary tract involvement and/or ureteric involvement, one is often impressed by the relative paucity of clinical and radiological evidence indicative of an outflow obstruction. We have all seen at cystoscopy in these cases a relatively normal prostatic urethra and bladder neck associated with a rather large atonic posteriorly displaced bladder base with angular, somewhat gaping ureteric orifices. Similarly, in the female child it is not uncommon to see what appears to be a very early stage of developing cystocele despite little evidence of any peripheral bladder neck or urethral obstruction. We have all had the feeling of irritation at our inability to unequivocally demonstrate a peripheral obstruction in these cases.

However, in the older age group a more clearly defined symptom complex will evolve. In the case of the male and particularly in the male in the third or fourth decade, a characteristic clinical picture is often found. This I choose to call the "male cystocele symptom complex." These people are characteristically tense, visceroptotic individuals, complaining of vague lower urinary tract symptoms (either infective or obstructive). They are often misdiagnosed as having chronic prostatitis, cowperitis, spastic colitis, or even proctitis. In the earlyst ages, they complain of hypogastric discomfort, intermittent mild obstructive symptoms of the urinary tract, and intermittent occasional bouts of frequency unrelated to any other urinary symptom; there is usually a history of recurrent treatment for chronic prostatitis stretching over a period of many years. In its later stages, this condition may be associated with more advanced obstructive and/or infective symptoms. Clinical and radiological examination may be singularly unrewarding, but at cystoscopy the appearance is quite characteristic.

There may or may not be overt evidence of a bladder neck contracture, but in all these cases, whether obstructive or not, there will be a rigid bladder neck. In the early stages, there will be a mild degree of elevation of the internal vesical orifice with a depressed bladder base, particularly behind the interureteric ridge. As the condition advances, this depression of the bladder base may reach such proportions that the bladder assumes the appearance of an inferior or infraposterior diverticulum. Associated with this is an atonic, large, dilated bladder with minimal evidence of trabeculation or hypertrophy of the trigone. (If these patients are exposed perineally, it becomes apparent that there is a complete divarication of the anterior portion of the levator ani and an almost nonexistent rectourethralis.)

It is important to note that this condition presents itself in virile, young, procreative males, and therefore it is of paramount importance that whatever is done to correct this state of affairs in these patients, the integrity of the internal vesical orifice and its ability to prevent reflux ejaculation must be preserved at all costs.

In the female, the condition is even more complex. We are aware that this condition can present itself in a number of different ways. Whereas there may be numerous precipitating factors dependent upon age or mental state, sexual relationship, pregnancy, infective foci, etc., it is still a truism that these patients would not be continually finding their way back to the urologist if it were not for the fact that there is a basic abnormality in the dynamics of their micturition. In the adult female, it often is apparent how easily these patients can be recognized on initially presenting themselves for examination. The asthenic, visceroptotic, emotionally labile and tense, postmenopausal female with a narrow subcostal angle, low-slung buttocks, and slightly convex but firm abdomen is the prototype.

The basic complaint is usually recurrent lower urinary tract infection, almost invariably associated with numerous other functional disturbances such as, for example, chronic constipation and/or spastic colitis. There is very often a previous history of gynecological surgery, most commonly vaginal hysterectomy and anterior colporrhaphy. On clinical examination, the findings are confined usually to the stigmata associated with acute or chronic infection.

Vaginal examination can, however, be of some assistance, and it is often possible to pick up salient features in these cases, namely, a broadening and posterior declination of the juxtacervical portion of the anterior vaginal wall, a marked posteroinferior angulation of the posterior urethrovesical angle, and a marked downward displacement of the pelvic floor with increased abdominal pressure.

SPECIAL INVESTIGATIONS

Apart from the routine radiological investigations, the following points are worthy of note:

The presence of a large, flaccid bladder in the nullipar is highly suspicious, particularly if there is a marked condensation of dye centrally located in the anteroposterior projection in the supine patient. This is suggestive of a deep posteroinferior *bas-fond.*

A direct lateral voiding cystogram using as a point of reference a line drawn from the inferior margin of the symphysis pubis to the middle of the body of the fifth sacral vertebra will serve to indicate the degree of displacement of the urethra relative to the pubis and the angulation of the bladder, using the bladder neck as the fulcrum.

Whereas the latter procedure will give us the opportunity of obtaining a permanent dynamic recording of a defect, panendoscopy of the over-distended bladder, to outline and fix the internal vesical orifice, will clinch the diagnosis, clearly demonstrating the acute angulation between the bladder and the urethra at the bladder neck, the marked posteroinferior displacement of the bladder base, the large atonic flaccid bladder wall, the absence of overt evidence of hypertrophy of the bladder wall, and evidence of persistent or previous infection. If the patient is asked to strain down as if to void, the marked downward displacement of the bladder base and angulation on the bladder neck can clearly be demonstrated.

In those patients in whom previous gynecological surgery has been performed, it is often possible to note a fixed rigid urethral floor associated with a bladder base which has been pulled posteriorly and fixed to the vault of the vagina.

It might be added that a similar situation can develop in the male after abdominoperineal resection because with total evisceration, of the pelvic intestinal contents, the large gap which is left, and the elimination of the supporting tissue to the bladder base will result in a marked posterior displacement of the bladder base and the vault into the floor of the abdominal pelvic pouch, and since the integrity of the pubovesical ligaments is maintained, an acute posterior angulation of the bladder on the bladder neck and the urethra occurs.

TREATMENT

The indications for repair of this situation are primarily those associated with any obstructive condition of the bladder in the male or the female. However, in those cases where there is basically a functional type of obstruction, it can often become extremely difficult, particularly where the young male patient presents with the symptoms of so-called recurrent chronic prostatitis and the female with chronic vesical irritation. In these cases when the patient often does not have an overt history of obstruction, the condition will be readily missed unless one has a high index of suspicion. A similar situation of course occurs with the young child, who is unable to differentiate the finer nuances associated with an obstructive bladder. It behoves us therefore to have a high index of suspicion as to this possibility in all cases of persistent or recurrent urinary tract infection with or without a history of previous pelvic surgery.

OPERATIVE MANAGEMENT

Operative management should be approached from two aspects. In the first place, it is often possible to prevent the development of this condition if it is borne in mind initially. Serious consideration must always be given to the immediate maintenance of a normal bladder position during and following pelvic surgery. However, where the condition has a developmental postural basis, or where the lesion develops postoperatively, the bladder displacement must be repaired. It may or may not be coupled with corrective plastic surgical repair to any outflow obstruction which may be present, such as, for example, a contracted bladder neck or prostatic hyperplasia, or with any anti-incontinence procedures, such as a urethropexy or a urethral sling procedure.

OPERATIVE PROCEDURE

After routine exposure of the prevesical space, the lateral endopelvic fascial space is developed down to the lateral aspects of the rectum or the vagina, as the case may be. Thereafter, the bladder is freed from its peritoneal attachment. This often requires some sharp dissection at the vault of the bladder around the urachus, but once this area has been dissected, one can reach very easily down to the vaginal vault or rectum along the postero-superior aspect of the bladder wall. In the female, it is possible to develop a plane between the bladder base and the anterior wall of the vagina as far forward as the bladder neck, identifying the ureters and the uterine artery and vein along the lateral aspects of the exposed area. In the male, a similar plane can be developed down to the entry of the ejaculatory ducts into the prostate. In both cases, it is possible to mobilize the bladder base and the trigone in its entirety and, as has been previously stated, to identify the ureters on both sides. In the female, after clearly outlining the anterior vaginal wall and fascia and the levator ani muscles on both sides, it is possible to repair any cystocele which may have been found preoperatively from this superior aspect.

After complete mobilization of the posterosuperior aspect of the bladder, and after particular care has been taken to completely free the lateral aspect of the bladder from the lateral endopelvic fascial space, it will be noted that a thick fascial layer, which is the extension of the pubovesical or pubocervical fascia, covers the posterosuperior aspect of the bladder wall.

Up to this point, the bladder has not yet been opened. This is now done through a V-shaped incision in the anterior bladder wall with the apex of the V situated over the bladder neck. In the elderly male patient, the obstructing prostatic tissue can now be visualized and routinely removed. In the younger male patient, no attempt whatever is made to interfere with the posterior vesical neck, but the trigone and bladder base are visualized and care is taken that all posteroinferior displacement of the bladder base has been eliminated by the previous dissection. The incision in the bladder is then extended to the proximal urethra in routine fashion, and anterior YV-plasty repair is completed. In the female patient with a history of stress incontinence, the previously mentioned procedures can be carried out at this stage as may be required. The whole bladder is rotated anterosuperiorly around the bladder neck and firmly attached to the periosteum of the pubis, or the rectus muscle fascia with nonabsorbable sutures. The retrovesical space and the bladder are drained in the usual fashion after closure of the wound.

In the female, care must be taken, if the vesical suspension is coupled with anterior YV-plasty, that the vertical incision into the dorsum of the proximal urethra is limited in extent, in view of the fact that there is a diminution of the urethrovesical angle as a result of the vesical suspension. It is important to maintain the normal urethrovesical angle while at the same time eliminating the obstructive element. An uncontrolled or overexuberant repair in this area might lead to stress incontinence. Apart from this, there are very few problems associated with this procedure. In the male patient, it has the advantage of complete reestablishment of a normal vesicourethral relationship, without in any way affecting the integrity of the bladder neck, particularly insofar as it affects the ejaculatory powers. It has the virtue that it in no way involves the trigone in any surgical intervention, thereby maintaining normal function of the trigonal muscle.

In the female, the procedure has a distinct advantage over anterior colporrhaphy as a method of management of cystocele. In the case of severe stress incontinence treated by urethropexy or a sling procedure, it has the added advantage that it tends to eliminated the sometimes distressing postoperative situation where in a patient has considerable difficulty in reestablishing normal voiding.

DISCUSSION

Although I am well aware that the factors I have mentioned are not necessarily the only factors involved in the etiology of recurrent urinary tract symptoms, I believe that it is important that we keep these factors in mind in the routine evaluation of these cases. Attention must always be directed toward determining whether a possible malassociation between the bladder and the urethra does in fact exist.

It is interesting to note that even up to the present day no satisfactory explanation for the occurrence of cystocele in the female[20] has ever been presented, and even less evidence has been presented to explain the development of this condition in the nulliparous. The high incidence of postoperative urinary tract infective and obstructive symptoms occurring after hysterectomy and other vaginal procedures in the female and after and abdominoperineal dissection in the male has been well documented[21]. Various premises have been advanced to explain this phenomenon[22]. Undoubtedly, some of these cases are due to impairment of the nerve supply to the bladder, or due to post-traumatic fibrosis and obstruction to the bladder outlet, or follow on chronic infective changes in the urethra after prolonged indwelling catheterization, but by far the majority of these cases do not present such overt evidence of disturbed vesical function.

If we further eliminate those patients whose symptoms are basically of psychosomatic or psychosexual nature, there remains a considerable number of cases, for which no satisfactory explanation could be found until our recent awareness of the role of functional obstruction to bladder outflow subsequent to postural changes in the vesicourethral unit.

Various authors noting a similar atonic nonovertly obstructed bladder occurring in young children presenting with recurrent urinary tract infection have sought to explain this condition as a vesical myopathy. On the basis of histological and histochemical changes noted in the bladder wall, they have sought to confirm a primary myopathic degeneration. I am, however, quite certain that these changes are perfectly compatible with any long-standing atonic dilatation of the bladder, with or without secondary inflammatory changes following on the infection, and do not represent a separate pathological entity.

Considering the role played by the trigonal muscle in the maintenance of the integrity of the ureterotrigonourethral unit as propounded by Hutch[16] and other workers, it is apparent that any alteration in the relationship between what Hutch chooses to call the "base plate of the bladder" and the vesical outlet will affect the functional integrity of the bladder. Therefore, in those cases where no satisfactory explanation for recurrent urinary tract infection can be found on the basis of accepted urological criteria, investigation and management as outlined above might be of value.

REFERENCES

1. Pierce, J. M., *et al.* Concept of resistance to flow applied to lower urinary tract. Surg. Gynec. Obstet, 116:217–222, 1963.
2. Falk, D. Treatment of resistant contracture of the bladder neck in women by plastic revision of the vesicle orifice. *J. Urol.* 79:447–552, 1958.
3. Folsom, A. I., and O'Brien, H. A. The female urethra—connecting links between urologist and gynecologist. *J.A.M.A.* 128:408–414, 1945.
4. Mckinnon, K. J., and Smith, E. C. Vesicle neck obstruction in women. *Can. Med. Assoc. J.* 71:356–360, 1954.
5. Emmett, J. L., Hutchins, S. P. R., and McDonald. J. R. Treatments of urinary retention in women by transurethral resection. *J. Urol.* 63:1031–1042, 1950.
6. Coutts, W. E., and Vargus-Zalazar, R. Acquired fibrosis of the bladder neck. *Brit. J. Urol.* 17:136–139, 1945.
7. Jacobson, C., Jr. Unrecognized vesical neck obstruction in women. *New Engl. J. Med.* 235:645–647, 1946.

8   Lintgen, C., and Herbult, P. Clinico-pathological study of 100 female urethras. *J. Urol.* **55**:298–300, 1946.

9. Mirabile, C. Resection of the bladder neck for obstruction in women. *New Engl. J. Med.* **228**:751–753, 1943.

10. Fister, G. M. Fibrosis and submucous calcification of the vesicle neck. *J.A.M.A.* **118**:604–606, 1942.

11. Folsom, A., and O'Brien, H. A. The female obstructing prostate. *J.A.M.A.* **121**:573–575, 1943.

12. Paquin, A. Urinary tract outflow resistance in normal human females. *Invest. Urol.* **1**:126–228, 1963.

13. Turner-Warwick, R. T., and Whiteside, C. G. Investigations of bladder outflow. *Mod. Trends Urol.* **3**:295–311, 1969.

14. Woodburn, A. T. Structure and function of the urinary bladder. *J. Urol.* **84**:79–85, 1960.

15. Collard, C. A., and Eastman, P. S. Urinary retention following combined abdomino-perineal resection. *Surgery* **14**:223–228, 1943.

16. Hutch, J. A. A new theory of the anatomy of the internal urinary sphincter and the physiology of micturition. *Invest. Urol.* **3**:36, 1965.

17. Gardener, S. A., *et al.* Cine and radiographic studies of female urinary incontinence. *Am. J. Obstet. Gynec.* **82**:112, 1961.

18. Karlson, S. Experimental studies on the functioning of the female urinary bladder and urethra. *Acta Obstet. Gynaec. Scand.* **32**:285, 1939.

19. Hunter, D. T. A new concept of urinary bladder musculature. *J. Urol.* **71**:695–704, 1954.

20. Warrel, D., and Scott, R. C. Investigation and treatment in over 200 complicated cases of urinary incontinence. *J. Obstet. Gynaec. Brit. Commonwealth* **122**:564–574, 1965.

21. Durfee, R. B. Anterior vaginal suspension operations for treatment of stress incontinence. *Am. J. Obstet.* **92**:610–736.

22. Shute, W. B. Vaginal support in stress incontinence. *Am. J. Obstet. Gynec.* **91**:824–836, 1965.

Angiographic Characteristics of Renal Hamartoma

Herbert Brendler* and John W. Maguire*

Albrecht([1]) in 1904 first coined the word "hamartoma" to designate a benign tumor in which there is abnormal mixing of the normal component tissues of the organ in which the tumor arises. Renal hamartomas are relatively uncommon and are frequently found in association with tuberous sclerosis. They can occur, however, as isolated entities. When associated with tuberous sclerosis, they are multiple and bilateral; if not associated with tuberous sclerosis, they occur as solitary lesions. These tumors contain variable amounts of fat, blood vessels, and muscles and are named accordingly: angiomyolipoma, myoangiolipoma, etc.

The following paper presents two cases of renal hamartoma recently treated at Mount Sinai Hospital. Special emphasis is placed on the angiographic findings. The first case was diagnosed preoperatively on the basis of characteristic angiographic findings. The second case demonstrates a previously undescribed angiographic characteristic of hamartoma.

CASE REPORTS

Case 1

B. R. (MSH No. 788011) was a 40-year-old female admitted in December 1969 for evaluation of a right renal mass. Three weeks prior to admission to the Mount Sinai Hospital, the patient entered another hospital because of severe right flank pain, fever, nausea, and vomiting. An intravenous pyelogram was made which showed a right upper pole mass (Fig. 1), and

*Department of Urology, The Mount Sinai Medical Center, New York, N.Y.

she was transferred to us for further evaluation. Physical examination revealed a well-developed, well-nourished female in no acute distress. There was no right costovertebral angle tenderness or palpable mass. Laboratory data: hemoglobin 9.9, hematocrit 29, white blood count 5000. The urine was acid, and there was no hematuria, pyuria, or proteinuria. SMA-12 values were all normal. Selective right renal angiography showed an upper pole mass with a central radiolucent area supplied by tumor-like vessels (Fig. 2). On the basis of these findings, a diagnosis of angiomyolipoma

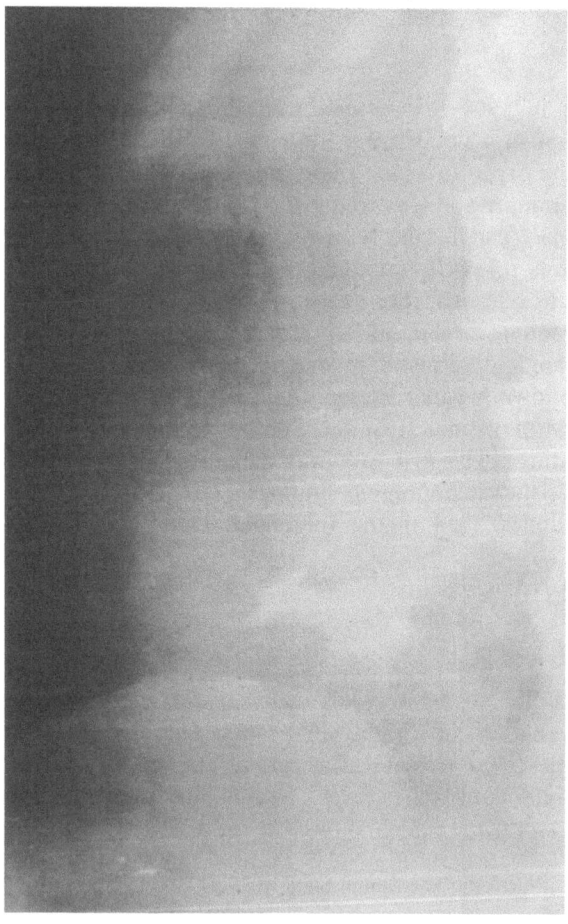

Fig. 1

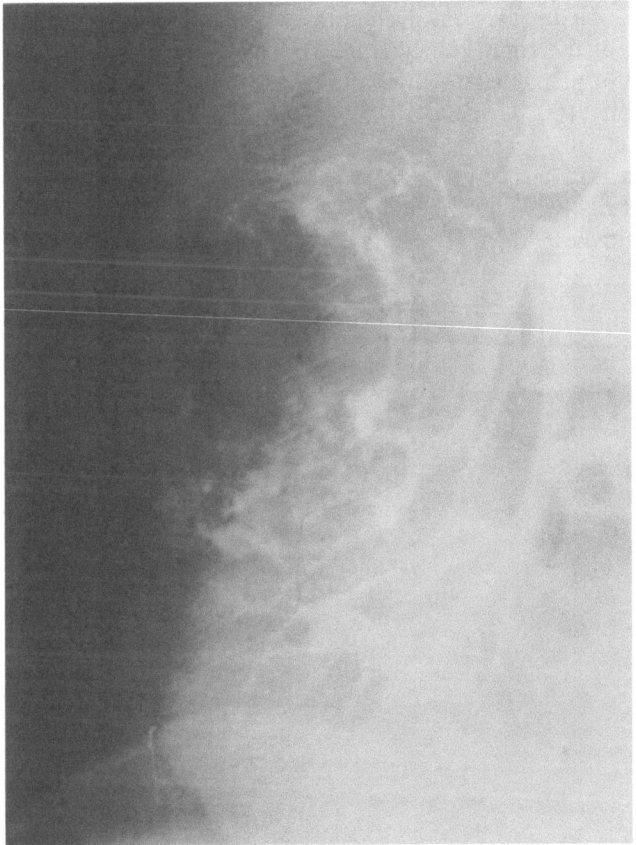

Fig. 2

was made. The patient subsequently underwent a right transperitoneal nephrectomy. The tumor was adherent to the vena cava and duodenum, from which it was dissected free. The patient received 3 units of blood during the operation; her postoperative hemoglobin was 11.1 She had a benign postoperative course and was discharged on the tenth postoperative day. Pathological evaluation revealed the tumor to be an angiomyolipoma with organized hematoma in a cystic cavity.

Case 2

L. U. (MSH No. 793937) was a 40-year-old female admitted for right renal mass. The patient was originally seen because of recurrent cystitis and hematuria. An intravenous pyelogram was made which showed an upper pole mass of the right kidney (Fig. 3). There was no costovertebral angle tenderness or palpable flank mass. Laboratory data: hemoglobin 13.3, white blood count 7400. Urinalysis showed rare red blood cells and occasional white blood cells. Urine culture was negative. SMA-12 readings were within normal limits. Chest X-ray and electrocardiogram were normal. The patient underwent right selective renal angiography. The first injection showed what appeared to be a normal angiographic pattern except for a small artery

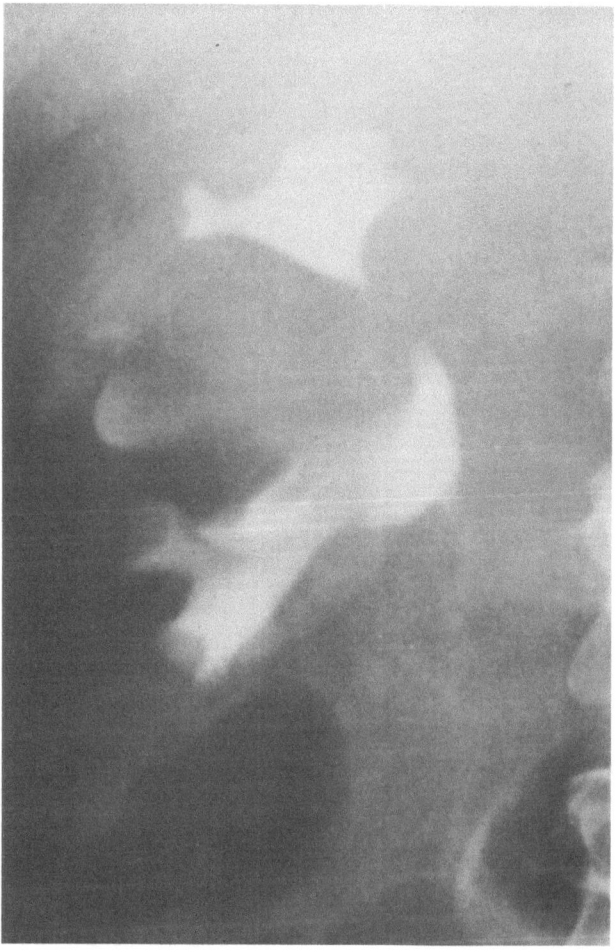

Fig. 3

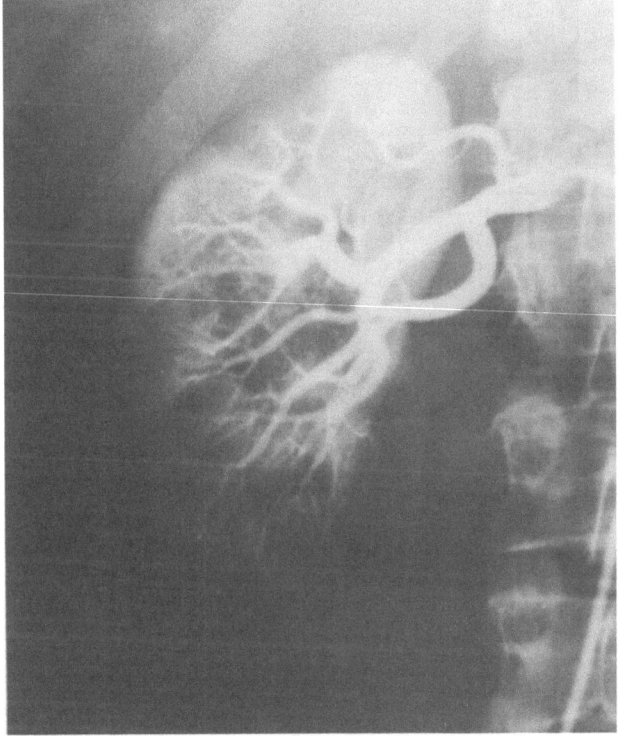

Fig. 4

in the upper pole resembling a tumor vessel (Fig. 4). The study was repeated with epinephrine injection, and this showed the characteristic vascular pattern of a renal neoplasm (Fig. 5). The patient underwent a right renal exploration. The external appearance of the kidney at the time of surgery was normal. However, because of the angiographic findings a nephrectomy was performed. The patient's postoperative course was benign. The pathological description of the tumor was angiomyolipoma.

DISCUSSION

The radiographic findings of renal hamartoma have received comparatively little attention in the urological literature. In 1961, the intravenous pyelographic findings of six patients with renal hamartoma treated at Mount Sinai Hospital over a period of 14 years were reported[2]. This tumor visualized typically as an intrarenal mass with distinct radiolucent areas.

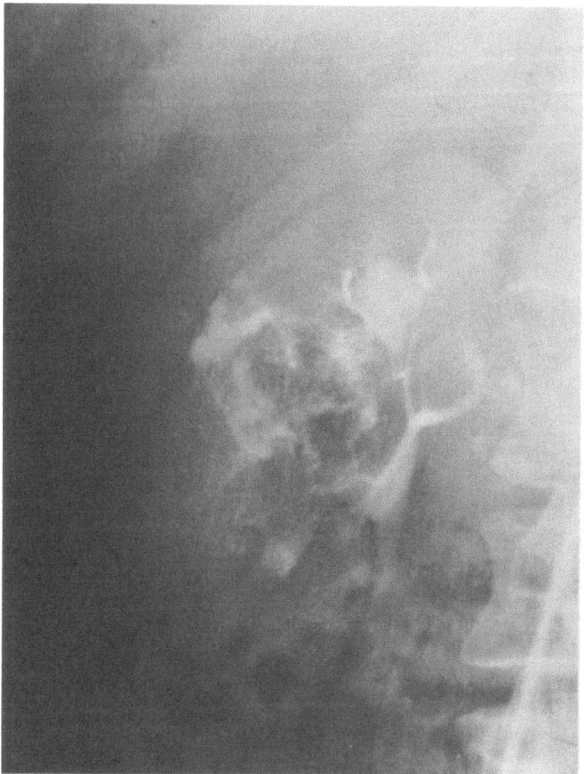

Fig. 5

These areas are thought to be due to the large amount of fatty tissue contained within them. The degree of lucency is less than that of bowel gas, but it
is often difficult to distinguish between the two.

The angiographic findings of renal hamartoma are of interest. The
mass visualizes well, as do the lucent zones seen on excretion urography.
Detailed examination of the vessels which supply the tumor shows them to
differ in certain aspects from those seen in renal cell carcinoma. They appear
dilated and tortuous, with many small branches, and they look sacculated,
with dye remaining in their saccules into the late venous phase[3]. In practice,
however, it may be difficult to distinguish the lesions from hypernephroma
solely on the basis of radiological appearance of the vessels. The first case
proved relatively straightforward in this respect because the radiological
criteria were easily satisfied, i.e., mass with lucent areas and vessels dem-
onstrably different than those seen in renal cell carcinoma (Fig. 2).

The second case is of special interest because of the lack of vascular response to epinephrine. The intravenous pyelogram showed a mass in the upper pole, but the angiogram showed a normal vascular pattern except for a small vessel which easily could have been missed (Fig. 4). The lack of response of the vasculature to epinephrine was identical with that seen in renal cell carcinoma, and this accounted for the preoperative diagnosis of hypernephroma (Fig. 5). The finding of a benign lesion at operation was entirely unexpected.

This case shows quite clearly that the lack of vascular response to epinephrine in a hamartoma can be indistinguishable from that in hypernephroma. Serial sections of the tumor showed no evidence of malignant change, either sarcomatous or carcinomatous, and so it may be assumed that the lack of epinephrine response is not necessarily an index of malignancy.

SUMMARY

Two cases of renal hamartoma are presented, with special emphasis on the angiographic findings. The first demonstrated the characteristic angiographic findings of hamartoma, i.e., a mass in the kidney with radiolucent areas supplied by tumor-like vessels. The second case was wrongly diagnosed preoperatively as a renal cell carcinoma on the failure of the tumor vessels to respond to epinephrine. This case demonstrates the fact that epinephrine response alone is not necessarily an index of malignancy.

REFERENCES

1. Albrecht, E. Über Hamartome. *Verh. Deutsch. Path. Ges.* 7:153, 1904.
2. Khilnani, M. T., and Wolf, B. S. Hamartolipoma of the kidney: Clinical and roentgen features. *Am. J. Roentgenol.* 86:830, 1961.
3. Khilnani, M. T., Abrams, R. M., and Beranbaum, E. R. Angiographic features of hamartoma of the kidney. *Radiology.* 90:999, 1968.

Recent Experiences at the Ochsner Clinic with Transureteroureterostomy

William Brannan*

The anastomosis of one ureter to the other as a definitive treatment for distal ureteral obstruction was first advocated by Sharp in 1906, using dogs and a cadaver as subjects. It was not until 1934, however, that the first clinical application was reported by Higgins[2]. Although successful, only five other cases had been reported by 1947, as physicians seemed reluctant to employ the technique either for fear of cross-contamination of the normal kidney by an infected one or for fear of obstruction at the site of the anastomosis.

During the past 20 years, only about 60 other cases have been reported in the *Journal of Urology,* although the success rate surpasses 95%. These reports have shown that the fear of injury to the uninvolved side is without foundation. Very few failures have occurred, provided the principles of plastic surgery were adhered to: namely, freedom from angulation, tension, and constriction, all of which compromise the circulation upon which the success of any surgical procedure depends. Stripping of the ureteral adventitia may also lead to necrosis. In the largest series thus reported, Hodges[3] describes only one technical failure out of 32 cases. This occurred when the transferred ureter pulled away under tension, resulting in a later nephrectomy on that side. However, it is of great importance that the contralateral upper tract remained normal, and the site of anastomosis closed as would any ureterotomy.

*Department of Urology, Ochsner Clinic and Ochsner Foundation Hospital, New Orleans, Louisiana.

METHOD

The technique as variously described is straightforward, and with an average degree of dexterity the results should be excellent.

In general, one first mobilizes a sufficient length of the diseased or damaged ureter to permit easy transfer across the midline and anastomosis to the opposite ureter. Care must be taken not to strip the adventitia of the ureter. A traumatized ureter should be resected up to a point of certain viability. Much more subtle is the ureter which has been included in a field of irradiation and which at a glance might appear normal—but on closer inspection could prove to be almost avascular near the distal end. A retroperitoneal tunnel is then dissected anterior to the great vessels in an area where the ureter can cross without angulation and cephalad to a point where there will be no tension. A longitudinal incision is made in the recipient ureter at this level. The distal 1.5 cm of the severed ureter is spatulated and sutured to the ureterotomy with 5-0 chromic catgut. Splinting is not necessary. The area is drained via a retroperitoneal Penrose drain brought out through a stab wound.

CASE REPORTS

Case 1

E. B. (No. 409692), a 7-year-old white female, was admitted with a history of three ureteroneocystostomies on the left, two on the right, and a bladder neck revision. Initial intravenous pyelogram revealed marked obstruction at the left ureterovesical junction with severe hydroureteronephrosis, and with essentially normal drainage on the right. Cystography failed to reveal reflux. An ileal conduit had been recommended elsewhere. A left nephrostomy was performed on August 22, 1969, with a subsequent left-to-right transureteroureterostomy on January 13, 1970. Follow-up intravenous pyelogram 2 weeks postoperatively, and at 3 and 8 months, revealed good bilateral drainage, and the child is still doing well at last report.

Case 2

J. M. (No. 400686), a 73-year-old white male, had the left lower one third of his ureter removed during an *en bloc* resection of the sigmoid colon for mucinous adenocarcinoma on October 24, 1968. Preoperative intravenous pyelogram on October 18, 1968, had revealed involvement of the left ureter with hydronephrosis on that side and bilateral renal stone disease in addition. A left-to-right transureteroureterostomy was done at the time of bowel resection. Follow-up intravenous pyelogram 5 weeks postoperatively revealed good bilateral drainage, but 1 week later a left renal stone descended and obstructed the left ureter, necessitating open removal, which was accomplished without difficulty on December 12, 1968. A final intravenous pyelogram on December 20, 1968, revealed no further obstruction. The patient continues to do well.

Case 3

D. M. (No. 409989), a 52-year-old white male, was admitted in February 1969 with a history of attempted left ureteral basket extraction of a lower one-third stone and inability to remove the basket. The patient was explored, the stone and basket were removed, and the ureter was splinted. Following splint removal, a stone which had been in the upper one-third of the ureter descended and obstructed at the same site, requiring a second open procedure. Postoperatively, the patient developed left flank pain. Admission intravenous pyelogram revealed left hydronephrosis and hydroureter down to a point 4–5 cm from the left ureterovesical junction. A left nephrostomy was performed initially on March 21, 1969, followed by a left-to-right transureteroureterostomy on May 29,1969. Follow-up intravenous pyelogram 9 months postoperatively was normal, and the patient continues to do well and the urine is sterile.

Case 4

S. L. (No. 718) was an 80-year-old white male with a 10-year history of recurrent bladder tumors. At age 76, a grade III transitional cell carcinoma of the bladder neck with muscle and prostate invasion was biopsied. He received 5400 rad to the bladder area. Subsequently, he had several transurethral resections and fulgurations of bleeding areas, and finally left ureteral obstruction was noted on intravenous pyelogram. A right-to-left transureteroureterostomy with a left skin ureterostomy was performed on October 30, 1969, for palliative urinary diversion. The patient lived 1 year, although an indwelling catheter was required to keep the ureterostomy from closing. The right kidney and total renal function remained normal during this time.

Case 5

L. J. (No. 701186), a 25-year-old Negro female, was admitted to the gynecology service with diagnosis of carcinoma, stage III, of the cervix with right ureteral obstruction. Following pelvic exenteration on August 15, 1969, a left-to-right transureteroureterostomy with skin ureterostomy was performed. An ileal loop was not performed because of the duration of the procedure and uncertainty as to her prognosis. She has been lost to follow-up, but an intravenous pyelogram 3 months postoperatively looked normal.

Case 6

C. A. (No. 117447), a 51-year-old white female, was admitted to the gynecology service with a left pelvic mass and left ureteral obstruction. At exploration on September 15, 1970, a 4–5 cm mass of endometriosis was found adhered to the left pelvic wall, ureter, and bladder. The left ureter was divided with as great a length as possible and transferred to the right ureter and anastomosed at a higher level. A current intravenous pyelogram reveals no hydronephrosis and good renal function bilaterally. She is asymptomatic with sterile urine.

Case 7

C. P. (No. 437007), a 50-year-old white married female, was admitted to the gynecology service on September 2, 1970, with a diagnosis of squamous cell carcinoma of the cervix, stage II-B, with post-irradiation 2 years previously. Examination showed extensive ulceration of the vaginal vault and cervix. Intravenous urograms and cystoscopy were normal.

On September 8, 1970, a Wertheim hysterectomy, pelvic lymphadenectomy, and excision of the upper one half of the vagina were carried out. At the time of surgery, both ureters were visualized and "stripped" but not otherwise damaged. The postoperative course was uneventful until the thirtieth postoperative day, when she began leaking urine from the vagina.

Urological examination disclosed a left vesicovaginal fistula with complete stenosis of the lower 2 cm of the left ureter. The bladder and the right ureter were normal cystoscopically and radiographically.

On October 15, 1970, a left-to-right transureteroureterostomy was carried out. The postoperative course was uneventful, and she was discharged on the twelfth postoperative day. She remains asymptomatic and has sterile urine without medication.

RESULTS

Seven patients have undergone transureteroureterostomy at this institution since October 1968. In each case there was either extensive scarring and fibrosis or tumor involving the lower one third of the pelvic ureter on one side with a normal opposite upper tract. Of the seven patients, five are living and asymptomatic relative to the urinary tract. One is lost to follow-up, and one has died of malignancy. Seven normal upper tracts have remained normal, and seven compromised upper tracts have been improved. In no case has there been extravasation at the site of anastomosis or subsequent obstruction. All urines have remained sterile, except in the one case requiring an indwelling catheter.

DISCUSSION

We believe that in cases where it is impossible or ill advised to reimplant a diseased or damaged ureter, it may be far safer and simpler to perform a transureteroureterostomy than to attempt other well-known methods of distal ureteral replacement, e.g., bladder flaps and ileal conduits. Our results, as well as those of all others reported, indicate that this procedure does not adversely affect a normal kidney or collecting system. It is more physiological than other methods and can often prevent a needless sacrifice of renal tissue.

In our two cases where one ureter was brought to the skin, we were anticipating future obstruction due to neoplasm in the pelvic area. Young[7] reports difficulty with the stoma of cutaneous ureterostomy and occasional slough of the longer ureter, which is frequently brought to the skin under some tension. Leakage at the site of anastomosis is also a concern when the longer ureter is under tension. However, there was no evidence of compromise of the function in the contralateral kidney in any of his 21 patients followed for more than 6 months.

SUMMARY

Seven patients underwent transureteroureterostomy. All had a good postoperative result insofar as preservation of function in both kidneys was concerned. There have been no deleterious effects on the contralateral normal upper tracts. We believe that this procedure should have a wider clinical application.

REFERENCES

1. Anderson, H. V. Transureteroureterostomy: Experimental and clinical experiences. *J. Urol.* **83**:593–601, 1960.
2. Higgins, C. C. Transureteroureteral anastomosis: Report of a clinical case *J. Urol.* **34**:349–355, 1935
3. Hodges, C. V. Clinical experiences with transureteroureterostomy. *J. Urol.* **90**:552–562, 1963.
4. Jacobs D., *et al.* Experiences with transureteroureterostomy. *J. Urol.* **97**:1013–1016, 1967.
5. Moore, T. D. Transureteropyeloplasty and transureteroureterostomy: The indications and operative technique. *J. Urol.* **60**:859–873, 1948.

6. Sharpe, W. W. Transureteroureteral anastomosis. *Am. Surg.* **44**:687–707, 1906.
7. Young, J. D., and Aledia, F. T. Further observations on flank ureterostomy and cutaneous transureteroureterostomy. *J. Urol.* **95**:327–333, 1966.

The Uses of Intestine in Urology (A "Gut Reaction," for W. W. S.)

Willard E. Goodwin*

The intestine, readily available to the urological surgeon as a substitute, as an isolated conduit, or as a closed system for urinary diversion, is an important and much used part of urological surgery. Most of the techniques we have learned and later employed were first worked out in the animal surgical laboratories, first in the laboratory of Professor W. W. Scott at the Brady Urological Institute, Johns Hopkins Hospital, Baltimore, and subsequently here at the University of California, Los Angeles.

In my view, each urological surgeon in training should have the benefit of this important and useful experience. I am grateful to Professor Scott for his thoughtfulness and understanding in providing this opportunity for me. Without it, my urological career would have been ordinary and undistinguished. With it *I have had the pleasure and excitement of exploring new horizons, in a new medical school. It is a life experience unparalleled in interest and opportunity.*

The various uses of intestine in urological surgery make up one of the most fascinating chapters in surgical history because of the many variations in technique and results. There is an immense literature on the subject, and

*Professor of Surgery, Urology (Pediatric), Department of Surgery/Urology, University of California School of Medicine, and the Wadsworth Veterans Administration Hospital, Los Angeles, California.

I shall here, chiefly, refer to some of my own contributions, each of which has its own bibliography.

URETEROCOLIC ANASTOMOSIS

It seems that the first urinary diversion to the bowel was by Simon, in 1851. Subsequent authors improved the technique by rolling the ureter between muscular flaps of bowel, but it was not until 1911 that Coffey's contribution ushered in the modern era of ureterointestinal anastomosis[1].

The best reviews of ureterocolostomy are by Hinman and Weyrauch[2] and by Nesbit[3].

Hudson, Cason, and I, working in Scott's laboratory, revived the Maydel–Bergenhem operation and subsequently employed it in some cases of exstrophy[4].

The late results of this procedure did not bear out our original enthusiasm, because many of the patients developed reflux and calculi, and most of them had to be converted to cutaneous diversion.

In 1947 and 1948, Harris and I, working in Scott's animal laboratory, perfected an *open, transcolonic* ureterointestinal anastomosis using a submucosal tunnel, very similar to that employed in ureterovesical anastomosis by the now eponymous Politano–Leadbetter method. This proved to be technically easy and seemed to be satisfactory when we tried it in dogs and monkeys. Subsequently, after my retransplantation to Califonia, I had an opportunity with Kaufman to employ this technique in a patient with carcinoma of the bladder, at the Wadsworth Veterans Hospital in 1952. The result was spectacularly satisfactory, and we have continued to use that technique for ureterosigmoid anastomosis since that time[5,6].

Although some authors have given up on ureterosigmoidostomy, and Stamey condemns it[7], I have continued to use it in selected cases. It is particularly suited to children with exstrophy of the urinary bladder, because it gives them a chance to grow up without an external appliance and with a socially acceptable external appearance. I also recommend it for young, vigorous people and pretty girls who need to have urinary diversion and do not wish to be encumbered with an external appliance. The perils of pyelonephritis and electrolyte imbalance need to be recognized and can be combatted by judicious use of antibacterial drugs and 10% sodium potassium citrate solution, plus a low chloride diet. If there is uncompromising deterioration after the operation, the situation is still recoverable by Bricker's cutaneous diversion or by diverting colostomy to provide a true rectal bladder[8,9]. Transureteroureterostomy may have a place as a valuable adjunct if one ureter begins to go bad while the other is perfect[10]. We have used this clinically in a few cases with satisfaction.

URETEROILEOCUTANEOUS ANASTOMOSIS (BRICKER'S OPERATION)

Bricker, in 1950, set the stage for the modern, much employed use of ureteroileocutaneous anastomosis[11,12]. This operation is probably the most widely used type of diversion and has made obsolete all other types of cutaneous urinary diversion, except when they are employed as emergency measures[13–15].

USE OF THE ILEOCAECAL SEGMENT

In cases where reconstruction of the urinary bladder and enlargement of its size seem indicated, the ileocaecal segment may be used with confidence of success. This procedure, popularized by Gil-Vernet, Jr.[16] is now being employed more and more in this country. Recently, we have had an opportunity to observe two patients who had this operation successfully performed here at UCLA by Gittes. One was a young boy with constant urination due to a small bladder, and the ohter was a teenage girl who had worn a suprapublic tube for most of her life. In each case, the urinary tract was rehabilitated to nearly normal by use of the ileocaecal segment to augment the size of the bladder and to make a conduit from the ureters to the bladder. The ileocaecal valve was employed to prevent reflux.

ILEOCYSTOPLASTY AND SIGMOIDOCYSTOPLASTY

Our own interests in augmentation of the bladder have centered around ileocystoplasty and sigmoidocystoplasty[17–24].

We have been generally satisfied with long-range results of ileocystoplasty, provided that proper indications were observed. Ideal candidates for enlargement of the bladder are those patients who have a contracted bladder due to interstitial cystitis, tuberculosis, or chemical injury.

At first, we employed both ileocystoplasty and sigmoidocystoplasty with about equal frequency. Unexpectedly, patients with ileocystoplasty seemed to have better results than those with sigmoidocystoplasty, in our hands. Without making an exact count, I would estimate that we have had approximately 50 experiences with ileocystoplasty. For the most part, results have been satisfying.

Enterocystoplasty should *not* be used for neurological bladders because of the problems with external sphincter spasm.

The most important consideration is to be certain to remove any vestige of lower urinary tract obstruction, and we now *always* employ a Y-V plasty type of operation on the bladder neck in both males and females whenever intestine is placed above the vesical outlet.

Our "cup patch" type of ileocystoplasty[20] has proved to be most satisfactory in our experience.

THE ILEAL URETER

One of the most interesting uses of intestine has been for replacement of the ureter[25-28]. One of the best recent reviews of the whole subject is by Lhez[29], which was originally presented to the French Urological Association.

We have used the ileum to replace the ureter in various circumstances where there has been surgical or traumatic loss of the ureter. One could think of it as Bricker's operation with anastomosis to the bladder instead of to the skin. It has been, usually, quite satisfactory, provided that the renal function was good and there was no outlet obstruction. If renal function is poor, or if there is outlet obstruction, the procedure is contraindicated.

One particular use of it has been in a selected group of patients who have recurrent multiple "staghorn" renal calculi[27]. The idea is to provide a new and wide-open conduit from the kidney to the bladder so that no further stones can form. Long-range results have justified cautious enthusiasm for this procedure in these selected cases. However, the operation will never become popular because it is so difficult and is reserved for those desperate patients who have had many previous operations for stone and who are poor surgical risks because of infection and recurrent calculi. The problems of postoperative infection and fistula, and of hemorrhage during the operation, have been extremely difficult in almost all cases. Nonetheless, we have had some remarkably successful results, even in patients with solitary kidneys, and I believe that the procedure can and should be used for properly selected patients who have multiple recurrent stones and who are unable, otherwise, to be stone free.

URETEROCOLONIC CUTANEOUS ANASTOMOSIS

In 1967, Mogg, of Cardiff, presented his technique and excellent results with the use of a conduit of sigmoid colon, instead of ileum, for cutaneous diversion[30]. His results and technique are excellent.

We have occasionally used this with great satisfaction. My first experience with it was in a child with exstrophy of the urinary bladder who had an incontinent anal sphincter as a result of an imperforate anus operation. The ureterocolocutaneous anastomosis was performed in 1952, and the child has grown to be a normal, healthy young man with the colonic diversion acting as well or better than diversion with ileum.

In a discussion of Smith's paper on Bricker's operation in 1958[31], I said the following: "There is no question that Bricker's operation is a valuable and important contribution to the armamentarium of the urological surgeon. There are occasional cases in which the same result may best be achieved by use of an isolated segment of a sigmoid colon. I should like to suggest that this always be borne in mind, *particularly in patients undergoing pelvic exenteration operations.* The feasibility of using the lower segment of the sigmoid colon for this purpose in a case of pelvic exenteration, with diverting colostomy above, should always be considered. Operation time is potentially reduced by the use of the already divided large bowel."

REFERENCES

1. Goodwin, W. E., and Martin, D. C. Commentary on "Physiologic implantation of the severea ureter or common bile duct into the intestine," by R. C. Coffey, M. D. In *Classical Articles in Urology,* Immergut, M. A. (ed.), Charles C Thomas, Publisher, Springfield, Ill. p. 306, 1967.
2. Hinman, F., and Weyrauch, H. M., Jr. A critical study of the different principles of surgery which have been used in uretero-intestinal implantation. *Trans. Am. Assoc. Genitourin. Surg.* 29:15–156, 1936.
3. Nesbit, R. M. Another hopeful look at ureterosigmoid anastomosis. *J. Urol.* 84:691–703, 1960.
4. Goodwin, W. E., and Hudson, P. B. Exstrophy of bladder treated by rectal transplantation of divided trigone. *Surg. Gynec. Obstet.* 93:331–342, 1951.
5. Goodwin, W. E., Harris, A. P., Kaufman, J. J., and Beal, J. J. Open, transcolonic ureterointestinal anastomosis, a new approach. *Surg. Gynec. Obstet.* 97:295–300, 1953.
6. Williams, D. F., Burkholder, G V., and Goodwin, W. E. Ureterosigmoidostomy: A 15-year experience. *J. Urol.* 101:168–170, 1969.
7. Stamey, T. A. The pathogenesis and implications of the electrolyte imblance in ureterosigmoidostomy. *Surg. Gynec. Obstet.* 103:736–758, 1956.
8. Goodwin, W. E., Ureterosigmoidostomy (open trans-colonic ureteral intestinal anastomosis). In *The Craft of Surgery,* Cooper, P. (ed.), Vol. 11, Little Brown and Company, Boston, Chap. 117, p. 1367, 1964.
9. Mathisen, W. *Clinical and Experimental Studies on Ureterocolic Anastomosis,* Oslo University Press, 1969.
10. Harbach, L. B., Kaufman, J. J., and Goodwin, W. E. Experiments in ureterosigmoidostomy: Transureteroureterostomy combined with ureterosigmoidostomy to allow a single ureterocolic anastomosis. *J. Urol.* 104:395–401, 1970.
11. Bricker, E. M. Bladder substitution after pelvic evisceration. *Sug. Clin. N. Am.* 30:1511, 1950.
12. Bricker, E. M. Commentary on Bricker's operation. In *Classical Articles in Urology,* Immergut, M. A. (ed.), Charles C Thomas, Publisher, Springfield, Ill. p. 319, 1967.
13. Bricker, E. M., Butcher, H. R., Jr., Sugg, W. L., and McAfee, C. A. Ileal conduit method of ureteral urinary diversion. *Ann. Surg.* 156:682–691, 1962.
14. Cordonnier, J. J., and Nicolai, C. N. An evaluation of the use of an isolated segment of ileum as a means of urinary diversion. *J. Urol.* 83:834–838, 1960.
15. Creevy, C. D. Renal complications after ileac diversion of the urine in non-neoplastic disorders. *J. Urol.* 83:394–397, 1960.
16. Gil-Vernet, J. M., Jr. The ileocolic segment in urologic surgery. *J. Urol.* 94:418–426, 1965.

17. Winter, C. C., and Goodwin, W. E. Cystoplasty to increase bladder capacity. Experimental use of isolated patches and loops of large and small bowel to increase urinary bladder capacity in animals. *Surg. Forum* **8**:646–649, 1957.
18. Goodwin, W. E., Turner, R. D., and Winter, C. C. Results of ileocystoplasty. *J. Urol.* **80**:461–466, 1958.
19. Winter, C. C., and Goodwin, W. E. Results of sigmoidocystoplasty. *J. Urol.* **80**:467–472, 1958.
20. Goodwin, W. E., Winter, C. C., and Barker, W. F. Cup-patch technique of ileocystoplasty for bladder enlargement or partial substitution. *Surg. Gynec. Obstet.* **108**:370–372, 1959.
21. Goodwin, W. E., and Winter, C. C. Technique of sigmoidocystoplasty. *Surg. Gynec. Obstet.* **108**:370–372, 1959.
22. Goodwin, W. E., Betenbaugh, H. S., Haynes. V. E., and Ross, S. C. Full-term pregnancy and spontaneous delivery after ileocystoplasty. *J.A.M.A.* **181**:906–908, 1962.
23. Goodwin. W. E. Ileocystoplasty. In *The Craft of Surgery,* Cooper, P. (ed.), Little, Brown and Company, Boston, Chap. 115, p. 1349, 1964.
24. Goodwin, W. E. Late complications of enterocystoplasty. *Acta Urol.* **37**:51–52, 1969.
25. Goodwin, W. E. Replacement of the ureter by small intestine. In *The Craft of Surgery,* Cooper, P. (ed.), Little, Brown and Company, Boston, Chap. 116, p. 1357. 1964.
26, Goodwin, W. E., Winter, C. C., and Turner, R. D. Replacement of the ureter by small intestine: Clinical application and results of the ileal ureter. *J. Urol.* **81**:406, 1959.
27. Goodwin, W. E., and Cockett, A. T. K. Surgical treatment of multiple, recurrent, branched, renal (staghorn) calculi by pyelo-nephro-ileo-vesical anastomosis. *Trans. Am. Assoc. Genitourin. Surg.* **52**:102, 1960.
28. Goodwin, W. E. Replacement of the ureter by small intestine—the ileal ureter. In *Modern Trends in Urology* (2ser.), Riches, E. (ed.), Butterworths, London, 1960.
29. Lhez, A. Les remplacements del'uretère, Masson et Cie, Paris, 1968.
30. Mogg, R. A. The treatment of urinary incontinence using the colonic conduit. *J. Urol.* **97**:684, 1967.
31. Goodwin, W. E. Discussion of paper by Smith, D. R., and Galante, M., "The use of the bricker operation in urology." *Am. J. Surg.* **96**:254 (Discussion, p. 262), 1958.

Relocation of Ureteroileostomy Stomata

Lester Persky*

The value of ureteroileostomy as an eminently satisfactory method for urinary diversion is attested to by the ever-increasing number of reports of its application to large numbers of patients. The indications, techniques, and complications of the operation have also been well documented[1-3]. Included in these various discussions have been references to stomal difficulties and their management[4]. In general, however, very little attention has been given to those infrequent situations in which actual replacement or relocation of the stomal site has been deemed necessary. In our own series this has been carried out in a small group of patients depending upon etiological factors, antecedent surgery, and underlying patient constitution.

MATERIAL AND METHODS

These situations necessitating total alteration have occurred altogether nine times in the management of over 500 patients with urinary diversion by ureteroileostomy cared for at the University Hospitals of Cleveland, Ohio, during the last two decades. The underlying disease processes for which ureteroileostomy has been done included neoplasm, exstrophy, a variety of neurological conditions, and, on occasion, incontinence secondary to trauma or previous genitourinary operative procedures.

The surgical approach in these revisions has in general been one in which we have attempted to mobilize the ileal segment by circumscribing the

*Department of Surgery, Division of Urology, Case Western Reserve University, and the University Hospitals of Cleveland, Ohio.

primary stomal site([5]) (Fig. 1). Though the original defect the length of ileum achieved is tunneled to a new location. Here a new rosette is formed, and the skin about the initial area is closed over the advanced ileum (category I). When this is not possible, and this technique is not applicable, actual formal laparotomy and the creation of a whole new abdominal opening are necessary (category II). In other instances, we have been able to work through the initial stomal site, and by utilizing blind, careful blunt dissection alongside the mobilized ileum, a totally new stoma has also been achieved successfully (category III). This technique has found usefulness in the treatment of ileostomies in general surgery([6]).

Our stomal routine in all three types of repair includes the excision of a button of skin, fascia, and peritoneum. The leading end of the stoma is everted with stitches placed between bowel edge, seromuscular coat, and subcutaneous tissue (Fig. 2). Representative cases corrected in each of these

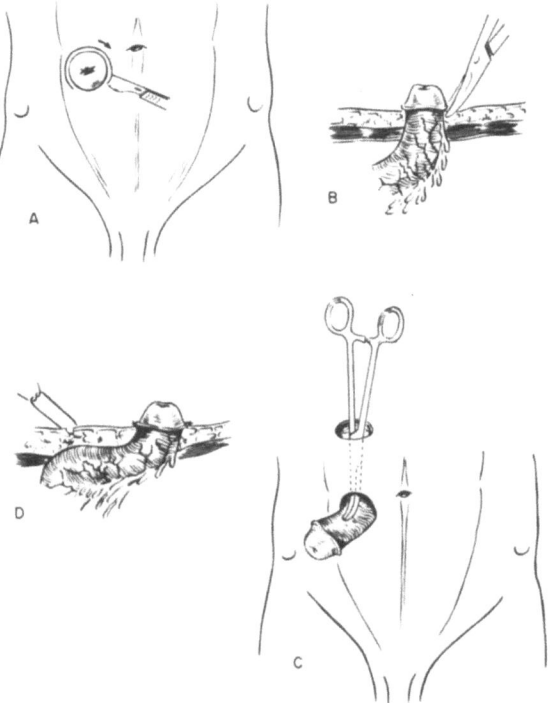

Fig. 1. Diagrammatic technique of relocating the stoma by freeing up the original area and tunneling it to a new site. The tunnel is placed subcutaneously and must rest easily without tension at its new location.

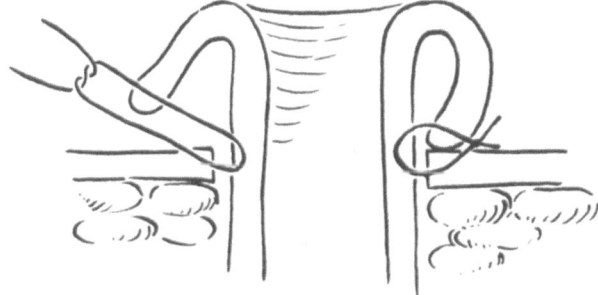

Fig. 2. Technique of forming an everted stoma. The stitches catch the leading edge of the ileum, the seromuscular, and the edge of the skin.

Table 1

Category	Description	No. of patients
I	Tunneling procedure	5
II	Formal laparotomy	2
III	Blind transperitoneal relocation	2

three fashions will be roughly summarized. Table 1 briefly outlines the number of patients in each of these treatment categories.

CASE REPORTS

Case 1, Category I

M. S. (No. 754–849) was a 13½-year-old white girl when first seen on the urology service in May 1964. She had been born with a congenital spinal cord injury causing paraplegia and incontinence of feces and urine. Recurrent urinary tract infections had been treated with long-term antibiotic therapy, and the blood woo nitrogen (BUN) had remained normal. She had had a bladder neck operation at age 3 and a pelvic laparotomy through a right transverse lower quadrant incision. Although she had a T-10 sensory level with spastic paraplegia, orthopedic procedures permitted her to walk with braces.

On physical examination she was bound to be a slightly obese but healthy appearing 13½-year-old girl with flabby abdominal musculature, a transverse right lower quadrant scar, and spastic paraplegia. BUN and serum creatinine were normal, with urine cultures yielding *Proteus*. Intravenous pyelography showed a small but functioning left kidney with clubbed calyces and a thick trabeculated bladder with multiple diverticula. On May 20, 1964, a bilateral end-to-side ureteroileostomy and incidental appendectomy were performed through a left paramedian incision with the stoma located in the right lower quadrant. Postoperative recovery was good.

After being free of fever on no medication, she was readmitted in February 1965 because of urine leakage around her ileostomy appliance at the location of the old transverse right lower quadrant scar. BUN, creatinine, cultures, and intravenous pyelogram were unchanged. To correct this urine leakage it was elected to move the stoma to the right upper quadrant, where it would be away from all old operative sites. This was accomplished on March 3, 1965, by means of a tunneling procedure, and the stoma has functioned well since. Yearly evaluation has shown no change in the BUN, serum creatinine, or urograms.

Case 2, Category II

J. R. (No. 813–867) was a 62-year-old short, heavyset, somewhat obese white male who presented in December 1964 with frequency and dysuria of several months' duration. He had had a partial cystectomy with placement of radon implants 10 months previously at another institution for transitional cell carcinoma of the bladder. This was followed by a transurethral resection of the prostate 2 months later. He had had an epigastric herniorrhaphy in the past.

He was a short, obese, elderly man with epigastric and suprapublic midline scars. Urinalysis showed microscopic hematuria. CBC, urine culture, blood chemistries, chest X-ray, liver scan, and bone survey were all normal. An electrocardiogram showed left axis deviation. The intravenous pyelogram showed normal upper tracts with a filling defect in the right lower bladder. On cystoscopy a tumor was seen which appeared to be infiltrating and involved the trigone near the right ureteral orifice.

Through a midline abdominal incision excising the previous scar, a cystoprostatectomy was done. No positive lymph nodes were found. After appendectomy, a conventional end-to-side ureteroileostomy was fashioned. The stoma was brought out in the right lower quadrant.

During the next several years he had a recurrence of his epigastric hernia twice, requiring repair, and a right inguinal hernia which had developed was repaired. He also had a large 10 by 10 cm ventral parastomal hernia which occurred in 1967 just below his ileal stoma in the right lower quadrant and was repaired through a curvilinear right lower quadrant incision.

Several months later, in March 1968, he was readmitted because the right lower quadrant ventral hernia recurred and was interfering with his ileostomy appliance. Because of this recurrent hernia and poor local tissue, it was elected to move the ileal stoma to a new location. Through a suprapubic midline incision made by excising the old scar, the ileal loop was freed up and moved to the left lower quadrant. The parastomal hernia was again repaired. He had an uneventful postoperative recovery, and his new stoma has continued to work well until the present.

Case 3, Category III

R. M. (No. 721–207) was a white female first seen in 1965 at age 8. She had been rendered paraplegic at delivery from birth trauma. Her brith had been a breech delivery with extraction forceps, and she sustained injury to the spinal cord at Cs with partial recovery. She was admitted for evaluation of urinary tract infection. She was a small, inactive child who had marked scoliosis, flabby abdominal musculature, and flaccid paraplegia with poor anal tone. Her upper extremities were weak but functional, and she could walk with leg braces and crutches. Severe scoliosis was still present. BUN was 10, and the urine grew a resistant strain of *E. coli*. Intravenous pyelography showed a small left kidney with decreased function and mild calyceal blunting on the right, and a large trabeculated bladder with significant residual. Cystoscopy confirmed these findings. There was no reflux on the cystogram, and cystometrics confirmed the diagnosis of neurogenic bladder with large capacity.

In October 1967 she was again admitted after several bouts of fever and pyuria. BUN and intravenous pyelogram were unchanged, but there was bilateral reflux on the cystogram. To protect her remaining nephrons, urinary diversion was planned. Through a left paramedian incision, bilateral ureteroileostomy and incidental appendectomy were performed. The stoma was placed in the right lower quadrant. The child had an uneventful postoperative recovery and was discharged.

Six months later, in early July 1968, she had a 3-day bout of nausea, vomiting, abdominal pain, and fever. At hospitalization, a rising BUN and serum creatinine and a nonfunctioning left kidney were found. On July 12, 1970, through a left paramedian incision because of possible extravasation, the ileal segment was revised with the stoma remaining at the original site in the right lower quadrant. The left kidney was excised because of nonfunction and repeated bouts of sepsis.

She was readmitted in September 1970 because of peristomal ulceration and scarring secondary to the trauma of her leg braces and urinary appliance.

BUN and creatinine were still normal, with unchanged creatinine clearance of the right kidney of 50 ml/min. On September 14, 1970, the old stoma was freed up and relocated in the right upper quadrant. This was done by blunt dissection through the original stomal site. The patient has continued to do well.

DISCUSSION

The difficulties attending stomal correction, epithelialization, and alteration have been described and are seen by all urologists managing these patients. Three of five patients in category I who were successfully manged by tunneling had these recurrent complications as the major cause of their need for complete stomal relocation. The other two patients had their repositioning forced upon us by our initially attempting to use the right lower quadrant when previous surgery had distorted the area. The two patients who had their reoperation done by formal laparotomy (category II) had the stoma shifted from the right lower quadrant to the left lower quadrant. This was forced upon us in one instance by a parastomal hernia which recurred after repair and seemed impossible to correct in any other way. The removal in the second patient in this category was necessitated by the attempt to locate the original stoma in the right lower quadrant, where marked distortion existed secondary to the correction of the abdominal wall defect attending exstrophy of the bladder (Fig. 3).

In the third category of reoperation we had two children. One of these children had marked peristomal ulceration due to the pressure of her drainage apparatus. Although the area healed with removal of the appliance, relocation seemed advisable since severe scarring had ensued. The second child had relocation necessitated by prior multiple incision in the process of creating a ventricular–peritoneal shunt at a very early age.

In these instances where more than mere local revision was necessary, a successful outcome uniformly eventuated. If we had been able to create a suitable subcutaneous tunnel of adequate length, this obviously would have been the method of choice. However, after multiple local attempts have failed, and where peristomal ulceration, scarring, and distortion have developed, we of course could not apply this effectively. We have learned now, after repeated failures, that prior disease in the anticipated area of appliance application should lead to seeking a more suitable primary site. Secondly, where there is going to be continuous need for braces, belts, splints, and supports of all types the abdomen should have a careful, preliminary surveillance with the anticipated stomal position and pressure of the appliance constantly in mind. Temporary testing and positioning of the drainage apparatus may be warranted prior to actual surgery, with daily

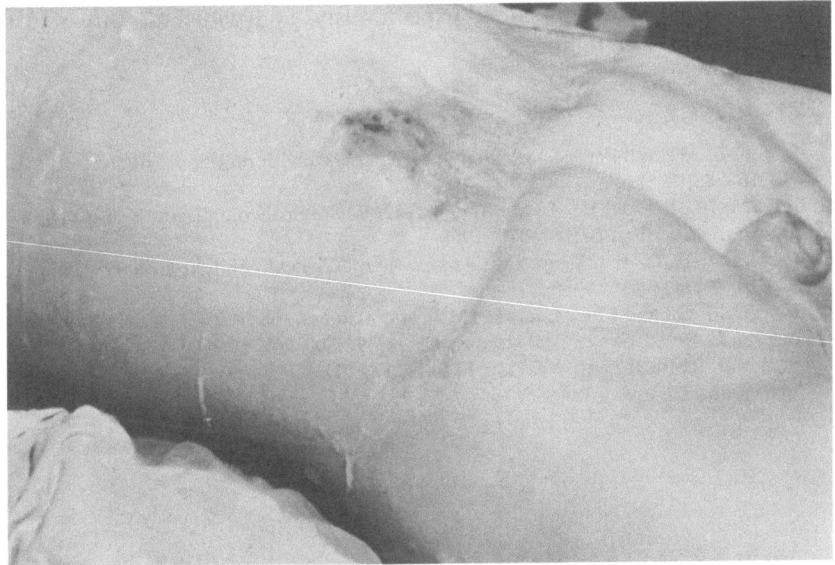

Fig. 3. Type of stomal location which leads to appliance failure, leakage, and patient discomfort. An alternative location should have been elected primarily.

activity as part of the evaluatory process. Thirdly, when advance total care of many of our myelomeningocele patients is being structured, consideration for possible late urinary diversion should preclude promiscuous abdominal incisions.

Although we have moved several of these new stomal sites from right lower quadrant to left lower quadrant, we have had no subsequent occurrence of intestinal obstruction. This may possibly reflect prior fixation of much of the intestine by adhesions. We are also very careful in doing the surgery to avoid narrow, possibly constricting spaces between the mesentery of the ileal segment and the abdominal parietes. When actual laparotomy has been necessary, we attempt to handle the remainder of the bowel as little as possible. Where we attempt the relocation blindly, so to speak (category III), we are careful to cease and desist if there is any impedance to gentle advancement of a probing finger or to ease of passing the ileal segment beneath the abdominal wall to the proposed new stomal location.

Although this experience with complete revision and resetting of the ureteroileostomy stoma and site has been a relatively small part of the management of these patients, it often has afforded us the greatest satisfaction in terms of happier patients, better loop function, more easily controlled appliances, and continued protection of upper urinary tract integrity. We feel that it can be done safely, expeditiously, and with little threat to the actual ureteral anastomoses.

REFERENCES

1. Cohen, S. M., and Persky, L. A ten-year experience with ureteroileostomy. *Arch. Surg.* **95**:278–283, 1967.
2. Jaffe, B. M., Bricker, E. M., and Butcher, H. R. Surgical complications of ileal segment division. *Ann. Surg.* **67**:367–376, 1968.
3. Parkhurst, E. C. Experiences with more than 500 ileal conduits in a 12-year period *J. Urol.* **99**:434–435, 1968.
4. Markland, C., and Flocks, R. H. The ileal conduit stoma. *J. Urol.* **95**:344–349, 1966.
5. Persky, L. Relocation of ileal stomas. *J. Urol.* **96**:702–703, 1966.
6. Turnbull, R. B., Jr., and Weakley, F. L. In *The Craft of Surgery,* Little, Cooper, P. (ed.), Brown and Company Boston. 1964.

Technique of Ileal Conduit—Evolution of the Brady Method

Lowell R. King*

It may seem presumptuous, and it may really be presumptuous, to write on the technique of ileal conduit surgery for an audience of highly trained urologists who competed successfully in an active residency training program and who have, as a group, pursued distinguished careers. On the other hand, though the mortality of the ileal conduit operation is below 2% in patients operated upon for benign disease, morbidity figures, particularly those reflecting long-term complications, remain quite variable. As an example, persistent infection is reported in some series in upward of 60% of conduits in patients with normal upper tracts. In my patients, this figure is about 10% in a comparable group. James Holland, reviewing "high" ileal conduits— those attached directly to the renal pelvis—found that only 40% remained infected in the postoperative period, a surprisingly good result when one considers that this form of diversion is elected most often in patients with extreme hydronephrosis([9]). These better results are probably directly related to operative technique and since the technique to be described, albeit with many digressions, evolved at Brady over the years 1955–1962, it seems a particularly apt subject for description and review in a Festschrift piece written to honor Dr. William W. Scott on his twenty-fifth anniversary as Chariman of the Division of Urolgy at Johns Hopkins.

*Department of Surgery, Division of Urology, The Children's Memorial Hospital, Chicago, Illinois, and the Department of Urology, Northwestern University Medical School, Chicago, Illinois.

THE ILEAL CONDUIT ARRIVES AT BRADY

The first ileal conduit at Johns Hopkins was performed in 1955 by Thomas Stamey, then chief resident. Prior to that, permanent diversion was performed by ureterosigmoidostomy, cutaneous ureterostomy, or permanent nephrostomy in patients requiring cystectomy for carcinoma of the bladder and by cystostomy, ureterostomy, or nephrostomy in those with hydronephrosis due to neurogenic bladder.

A review of the patients undergoing cystectomy for bladder cancer during the years 1930–1952 revealed that only 15 of 71 patients had survived longer than 5 years; 13 clearly died of the complications of diversion rather than their tumor, and many more experienced serious morbidity. The only patient to survive for more than 15 years was an old lady, living in a nursing home, with a permanent nephrostomy. Those who did not die of recurrent carcinoma died of the complications of the diversions listed above. Though the result of diversion in patients with hydronephrosis secondary to neurogenic bladder during a comparable period has not, to my knowledge, been reviewed, I think it is safe to say that few long-term survivals were achieved. These tragic results occurred in spite of great attention to technique. Ireterosigmoidostomy, all but given up by 1955, was performed only when the ureters were implanted into the sigmoid by an "antireflux" technique worked out by Dr. Jewett in 1941(²). In retrospect, perhaps mucosa-to-mucosa anastomoses, using more delicate suture material, would have had a favorable effect on results. As I recall, postoperative problems were usually due to obstruction at the site of ureteral implantation.

Good results were achieved by cutaneous ureterostomy only when the ureter was dilated. Even in such instances, stomal slough, and subsequent stenosis, often dictated permanent intubation or conversion to nephrostomy. Though stomal problems were at times caused by devascularization of the ureter during mobilization, it seems, again in retrospect, that the common stomal infarctions were due to the technique of forming the stoma. A stab wound was made in the abdominal wall, and the ureter was drawn through this. No effort was made to excise a "plug" of abdominal wall to allow the ureter free egress without constriction. This maneuver, a latter-day feedback from ileal conduit surgery, has made ureterostomy much more reliable, and the procedure is enjoying a deserved renaissance. In 1955, progressive stomal edema, impairment of venous drainage, and then arterial compromise and slough were almost the rule.

This was the context in which the ileal conduit arrived at Johns Hopkins, and the time was ripe. At first, Dr. Stamey closely followed the technique outlined in 1955 by Justin Cordonnier(³). I do not remember if the "corkbore" incision in the right lower quadrant for the exit of the distal end of the loop was made prior to opening the abdomen in the first few cases, but in general this was not done. Great attention was paid to trying to hold the wound edge in normal anatomical position when this incision was made later in the operation. An early patient, I believe the sixth in the series, died of postoperative obstruction at the site of ureteroenterostomy and consequent pyelonephritis. For this reason, when the ureters were of normal caliber, they were identified and ligated at the lower third early in the procedure. The ureters were then somewhat dilated by the time they were anastomosed to the ileal conduit, facilitating a precise anastomosis which was carried out using one layer of interrupted chromic catgut sutures, usually 4–0 in caliber. These sutures were placed with the knots outside the anastomotic lumen, since it was apparent that the knots of five or six sutures, the number generally employed, could obstruct the lumen of a ureter of normal caliber.

Stamey's and Scott's publication, in 1957, of the technique of ileal conduit surgery was based on 11 cases and was a milestone in the development of this operative procedure([4]). The drawings from his article are reproduced as Fig. 1. The salient points of the technique were as follows:

A bowel prep was usually employed.

1. The abdomen was opened through a midline incision, skirting the umbilicus to the left, to preserve the integrity of the skin of the right lower quadrant where the stoma, and appliance, would be placed. A left paramedian incision served as well.

2. The ureters were first identified and exposed by incision of the overlying posterior parietal peritoneum. They were tagged with umbilical tapes, or transected close to the bladder, and, in the case of ureters of normal caliber, ligated. The left ureter was most easily exposed by reflecting the sigmoid medially, opening the peritoneal reflection in the paracolic gutter. The ureter was seen as it was elevated, adherent to peritoneum, or plapated crossing the ileac artery. The left ureter was transposed, retroperitoneally, under the sigmoid when it was to be anastomosed to the ileal loop.

3. A segment of ileum, generally about 20–25 cm in length, which was supplied by at least two radial intestinal arteries, was then selected for the conduit. The mesentery was often transilluminated if the vessels were not readily visible.

4. Radial mesenteric incisions were made at either end of the selected loop. Isoperistaltic orientation was maintained by tagging the distal end of the conduit with a silk suture, held long, while a short suture was used to mark the proximal end. The mesenteric incisions were made to a depth of about 5 cm, dividing the vessels along the edge of the mesentery and cleaning the mesenteric border of the ileum of fat to facilitate accurate ileoileostomy. All mesenteric vessels were tied with silk, usually after each vessel was divided. Extreme care was used to prevent mesenteric hematoma.

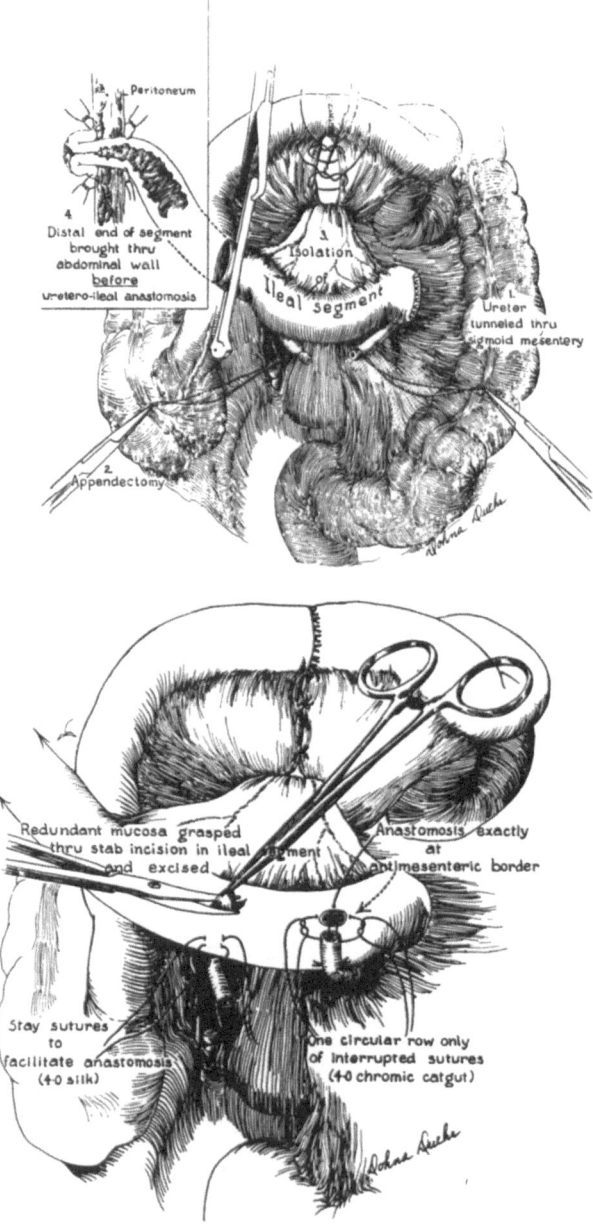

Fig. 1. Illustrations from Stamey's and Scott's article[4] detailing the technique of ileal conduit construction. This technique is discussed in the text. (Reprinted with the permission of *Surgery, Gynecology, and Obstetrics*.)

5. The ileum was then divided between Kocher clamps, at either end of the loop. Noncrushing rubber-shod clamps were placed on the small bowel above and below the site of reanastomosis to prevent leakage of bowel content. The conduit, protected by wet saline pads, was then dropped inferiorly against the sacral promontory, and continuity of the intestine was restored by ileoileostomy. A strict Halsted technique was employed in the bowel reanastomosis. The serosa of the posterior wall of the bowel was reapproximated with interrupted 4–0 silk sutures. The end sutures were held long. The bowel was then turned 180 degrees with these, and the Kocher clamps were removed. Crushed tissue was excised, and bleeding points were ligated with 4–0 plain gut. The bowel edges were then reapproximated with two running 4–0 or 5–0 plain catgut sutures, placed through full thickness of the ileum by the "over-and-over" technique along the back wall and using a Connell technique on the front to avoid narrowing the lumen of the a-nastomosis. A front layer of Lembert–Halsted interrupted silk sutures completed the anastomosis inverting the mucosal edges. The rubber-shod clamps were removed, and the lumen was checked for patency. This technique was very reliable when carefully done.

6. The mesenteric edges were approximated with interrupted 4–0 silk sutures, taking care not to puncture blood vessels running near the edges.

7. The appendix was removed, so that the cecum need not be manipulated after the ileostomy stoma had been formed. This could also be done earlier in the procedure.

8. The distal end of the isolated ileal segment was led out through a "cork-bore" incision in the right lower quadrant, just at or above McBurney's point, from which a circular "plug" of all layers of the abdominal wall had been excised. The defect was similar in diameter to that of the ileum, or slightly larger. In the original technique the stoma was formed with a single layer of interrupted 3–0 chromic sutures placed through the skin edge, the serosa of the bowel about $2\frac{1}{2}$ cm proximal to the end, and all layers of the bowel wall at the edge. When tied, these sutures everted a nipple that stood $1-1\frac{1}{2}$ cm above skin level, which aided the patient in positioning the appliance.

9. The proximal end of the conduit was closed in two layers—first with a running suture of chromic catgut and then with interrupted Lembert–Halsted serosal sutures to invert the closed bowel edges.

10. Ureteroenterostomy was carried out in a standard fashion. First, two 4–0 silk sutures were placed between the serosa of the midposterior bowel wall and the adventitia of the rureter $1-1\frac{1}{2}$ cm above the level of the projected anastomosis, which was placed at the antimesenteric border of the bowel. These sutures were tied and held, stabilizing the anastomotic site. The ureter was then transected obliquely opposite the anticipated point of

ureteroenterostomy, and this was where a small opening was carefully enlarged to correspond to the ureter in diameter. Anastomosis was carried out by placing interrupted 4–0 sutures through all layers of ureter and bowel wall. The bites were small and perhaps 1–2 mm behind the mucosal edges. The posterior sutures were placed first and tied; the anterior sutures were held until all were in to facilitate good visualization while the last were being placed. Either ureter could be done first; the left was frequently drawn under the sigmoid and anastomosed before the right.

    11.   A Levine tube was inserted and palpated in the stomach to ascertain good position, and the abdomen was closed by any of several acceptable techniques.

King and Scott[5] reviewed 83 patients operated upon using this technique in 1960; four had died in the immediate postoperative period, for an intraoperative mortality rate of 4.8%, certainly not excessive for patients undergoing ileal conduit in the years 1955–1960, and not excessive today when one considers that nearly half these diversions were done in patients with bladder cancer. These operations were performed 7–10 days prior to cystectomy, concomitant with cystectomy (performed by the same surgeon), or for palliation. When employed in patients with benign disease (neurogenic bladder, exstrophy, etc.), the bladder was usually not removed.

Several interesting facts did come to light in these early years, noted in the review of the first 83 patients[5]. When an intravenous pyelogram was obtained in the immediate postoperative period, upper tracts which had been normal prior to diversion usually exhibited some degree of dilatation. This was more often true of the left kidney and ureter than the right collecting system. This finding was attributed to the effect of higher ureterolysis on the left side, done in order to pass the left ureter under the sigmoid. Review of long-term results, however, revealed that persistent left hydronephrosis was also more common than right-sided dilatation (again, in patients with normal upper tracts prior to surgery). At reexploration, this was found usually to be due to sharp angulation of the left ureter as it passed under the colon, caused by a sizable blood vessel, usually an artery, and led to a refinement of technique. Left ureterolysis was carried even more rostral, often to the lower pole of the kidney, and the ureter was then passed beneath the large bowel posterior to the inferior mesenteric artery and branches in the sigmoid mesentery. More care was exercised to see that the ureter ran to the conduit implantation site in a smooth curve, especially in this region.

Other complications, both short and long-term, were noted. Urine leaks into the abdomen and through the major incision occurred from the site of ureteroileostomy in four patients. Three of these, with sterile urine, sealed spontaneously, though the leaking anastomosis eventually strictured, necessitating later repeat ureteroenterostomy. The fourth patient, with infected urine, developed peritonitis and died. For these reasons, urine leaks from the ureteroenterostomy are now treated as emergencies when the urine is known to be infected. Immediate repeat laparotomy and revision of the anastomosis is the treatment of choice, though nephrostomy is occasionally safer, especially when the leak becomes apparent after the fourth postoperative day. Patients with a leak and sterile urine may safely be watched for 48 hr—revision of the anastomosis is elected if the urinary drainage from the wound does not stop within this period of time.

Major problems were encountered in stomal management. Peristomal hernia occurred in two of 83 patients in the immediate postoperative period. Four more were encountered which occurred within 2 years of diversion. Hyperkeratosis of the stoma caused by squamous metaplasia of the bowel mucosa, leading to stricture, residual urine in the loop, and infection, was an even greater problem.

It seemed that eversion of the ileal bud to an elevation of more than 1 cm above skin level clearly predisposed to trauma, bleeding from the bud, and perhaps irritation leading to hyperkeratosis. This impression was reinforced when we found that the incidence of troublesome metaplasia was greatly reduced when an all-plastic, rather than rubber, collecting device was employed. These observations led us to form a flush or only slightly everted stoma and to finish the ileostomy with more care to prevent hernia.

Although the patients in this series were not carefully reviewed to ascertain the incidence of infection after diversion, it became clear that excessive conduit lengths predispose to stasis and infection. This stimulated the use of a shorter length of ileum for the conduit. The technique presently employed is described below and illustrated in Fig. 2.

The most common problems occur at the stomal site, one of which is obstruction by fascial baffles. This can be avoided by making the ileostomy incision before the abdomen is opened, as advocated by Cordonnier. A "cork-bore" plug of all layers of the abdominal wall is excised. The abdomen is then opened through a midline incision, skirting the umbilicus to the left, or through a left paramedian incision. The peritoneum is explored, and appendectomy is performed. The ureters are then identified; the right can usually be visualized through the posterior parietal peritoneum or can be palpated against the underlying ileac artery. The ureter is dissected inferiorly to the bladder and is surrounded by an umbilical tape for easy retrieval. The sigmoid colon is then reflected medially, and the lateral peritoneal reflection is opened. The left ureter is usually elevated with the peritoneum and is readily identified. It is dissected inferiorly to the bladder and is also mobilized superiorlly to the lower pole of the kidney. The upper left ureter requires this superior mobilization so that it can later be drawn under the sigmoid in

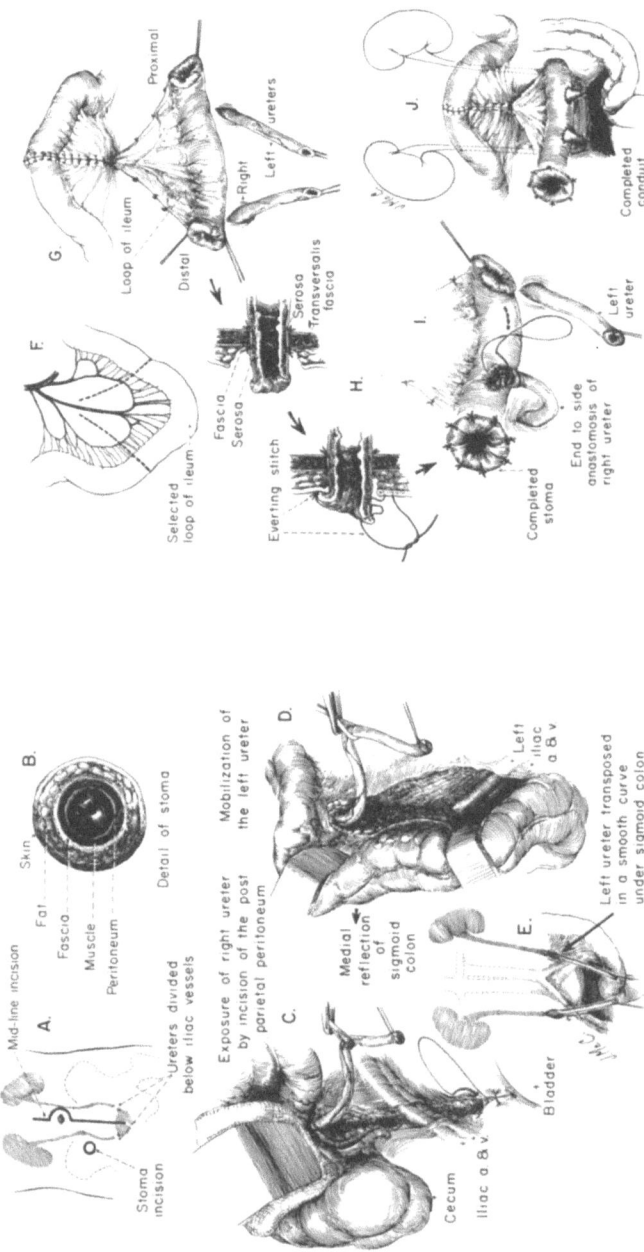

Fig. 2. The technique of conventional ileal conduit presently employed. A: Sites of incisions. B: Detail of "cork-bore" incision at stoma site. C: Mobilization of right ureter necessary to prevent angulation by the posterior parietal peritoneum. D: Exposure of left ureter. E: Left ureter transposed under sigmoid mesentery. F: Selection of conduit. G: Isolation of conduit and ileal anastomosis. H: Maturing stoma with slight eversion to aid in positioning appliance. Note fascial stitches, necessary to prevent hernia. I: One layer ureteral anastomoses. J: The completed loop. Any excess bowel proximal to the site of left ureteral implantation is resected before the proximal end is closed.

a smooth curve, without angulation. The left ureter is also taped for easy retrieval.

Attention is then turned to selecting a suitable segment of ileum to serve as the conduit. The terminal ileum is preferred for a conventional conduit, as the mesentery is usually deepest at this point, and a definite vascular arcade formed by two major vessels often supplies a loop of suitable length. In any case, a segment 20–22 cm in length, supplied by at least two radial arteries after division of the mesentery, is selected. The distal end of the proposed isolated segment is tagged with a long suture to help in maintaining isoperistaltic orientation. The mesentery at the distal end of the loop is then incised radially to a depth of 6 cm; the proximal mesentery need be incised to a depth of only approximately 3 cm. The mesenteric border of the bowel at the sites of transection is carefully cleaned over a 1–2 cm length to facilitate reanastomosis. Two matching Kocher clamps are applied to the bowel at either end of the prepared loop. The clamps are angulated so that the bowel is transected slightly obliquely. This ensures a good blood supply to the antimesenteric border of the ileum at the site of reanastomosis and increases the area of the anastomotic lumen.

The bowel is divided between each set of clamps. The loop so isolated is wrapped in a saline sponge and dropped against the sacrum. Intestinal continuity is re-established ventral to the isolated loop. I prefer a two-layer anastomosis, using a running 4-0 or 5-0 chromic catgut suture through the full thickness of the bowel wall, locking every other stitch to prevent bunching, on the posterior layer, and a Connell-type locking and inverting stitch for the anterior wall; however, a one-layer interrupted silk closure is being employed by many, and seems to serve as well. The anastomosis is then reinforced, and the primary anastomosis is inverted by a layer of 4-0 silk Lembert–Halsted sutures. The anastomosis is checked for patency, and the mesenteric leaves are approximated with interrupted 4-0 silk sutures to prevent internal hernia.

Attention is then turned to the ileal conduit. The stoma is finished first. The distal end of the isolated bowel segment is led outside the abdomen through the circular incision which was made before the abdomen was opened. This is usually in the right lower quadrant, centered just above McBurney's point, but may be in the belt line on the right upper quadrant when old scars, skin folds, or scoliosis have made the abdominal wall irregular at the usual site.

A three-layer anastomosis is necessary to prevent parastomal hernia. Six or eight interrupted 3-0 or 4-0 silk sutures are used to approximate the peritoneum–transversalis fascia and the external oblique–anterior rectus fascia to bowel serosa in separate layers. Three-zero chromic catgut is used to suture skin to the full thickness of the transected distal end of the conduit.

The serosa is usually picked up about 1 cm behind the end of the loop with this stitch. When tied, this everts the bowel mucosa slightly, forming a raised bud which aids the patient in positioning the appliance.

The right ureter is next reidentified and transected near the bladder. The distal stump is tied or suture-ligated. A traction suture is placed through the end of the ureter, which is then drawn against the antimesenteric border of the conduit. It is ascertained that the right ureter is not angulated by the posterior parietal peritoneum where it passes ventrally to meet the loop. The peritoneum covering the ureter may require further incision rostrally to permit the ureter to run to the loop in a smooth curve. Two silk sutures are then used to approximate the ureter to the posterior wall of the isolated loop about a centimeter above the site of anastomosis. These are placed through ureteral adventitia only, and are tied and held. This stabilizes the area of anastomosis.

A small incision is made in the bowel at the antimesenteric border, opposite the ureter. This opening is enlarged until it is slightly larger than the ureter to be anastomosed. The ureter is then transected tangentially to increase the area of the anastomosis. The full thickness of the ureter is then approximated to full thickness of the bowel with interrupted 5-0 chromic sutures. Six sutures are usually employed when the ureter is of normal caliber. All knots are outside of the lumen of the anastomosis. The most dorsal sutures are placed first and are tied when placed, whereas the ventral sutures are held untied until all have been placed. This facilitates accurate placement of the final sutures. After all have been tied, the silk retention sutures are cut.

No attempt is made to perform ureteroenterostomy by an antireflux technique. If the loop functions properly, that is, as a conduit, the lumen will be wet, but urine will not be retained in the loop. Reflux therefore will not occur unless the stoma is occluded, as for an ileogram. When this type of X-ray is performed, eight of ten of the ureters reimplanted in this manner will show reflux. This is sometimes an aid in delineating the upper tract after diversion.

The left ureter is implanted in like manner. More care must be taken on the left side to see that the ureter is not angulated by the inferior mesenteric artery, or its branches, as it passes beneath the sigmoid mesentery. The transected left ureter should pass from the lower pole of the kidney under the sigmoid and into the peritoneum over the sacral promontory in a smooth curve—almost a straight line. The implantation site on the loop is usually 2-3 cm proximal to the site of the right ureteral anastomosis.

Excessive length of the blind end of the conduit is then resected. This prevents pooling of urine, which may be a cause of infection. This maneuver, closing the proximal end last, was suggested by Dr. Paul H. Good. Closure is usually accomplished in two layers—first a running 4-0 chromic suture through all layers of the bowel and then a layer of 4–0 silk Lembert–Halsted sutures to invert the catgut closure.

Rents in the peritoneum are closed, and a nasogastric tube is inserted and palpated in the stomach to ascertain its position. All anastomoses are checked for patency. Indigo carmen may be given intravenously to check for leaks at the ureteroileal anastomosis, or the loop may be distended with sterile saline injected by asepto syringe through the stoma (another of Dr. Good's innovations, as I recall). The abdomen is closed layer by layer. I usually employ heavy retention sutures, placed through all layers of the abdominal wall except peritoneum, to guard against wound dehiscence in patients with neurogenic disease and those undergoing cystectomy simultaneous with urinary diversion. In other instances, the pull-out retention sutures are omitted.

Where a paramedian incision has been employed, each fascial layer is closed with interrupted silk sutures. Since a midline incision presents only one fascial layer for closure, wire sutures are usually elected. A temporary ileostomy appliance is fitted in the operating room. A good fit can be achieved while the patient is still anesthetized, and the wound is kept dry in the vital first few hours so that it can seal without an added risk of bacterial inoculation.

THE CASE FOR TOTAL URETERAL BYPASS BY PYELOILEAL OR PYELOJEJUNAL CUTANEOUS ANASTOMOSIS

Patients with marked hydronephrosis, usually children with neurogenic bladder or (closed) exstrophy, were found often to do poorly after ileal conduit performed in the manner outlined above. Of 15 kidneys (renal units) rated as markedly dilated at the time of diversion, 12 worsened subsequently[5]. When hydronephrosis in children was mild, only four of 16 deteriorated further during follow-up. Some of these patients might now be considered good candidates for cutaneous ureterostomy; at the time (1958), the problem was resolved in another manner.

The etiology of the progressive hydronephrosis in the absence of demonstrable obstruction in the diverted urinary tract was thought to be absence of effective peristalsis in the hydronephrotic ureteral segment proximal to the ileal loop. Whether this is, in fact, a significant factor is still, I think, unproven. Renal function in dogs remains stable when ureteral peristalsis is ablated[6]. Many patients with ureteral dilatation to a degree preventing coaptation of the walls and closure of the lumen—necessary to produce intraluminal pressure changes—do quite well when followed over a period of many years if such dilatation is not due to obstruction. In other instances, obstructed dilated ureters may do very well after removal of the obstruction, or subsequent to ureterostomy, even though effective peristalsis never returns. However, to the best of my recollection, loss of peristalsis was our working hypothesis to explain progressive hydronephrosis after diversion in these patients, and it was in this context that Dr. Fredrick Burt applied his genius to the problem.

By 1958, four "ileal ureters," employing an isoperistaltic ileal segment to conduct urine from renal pelvis to bladder had been tried at Johns Hopkins; none were successful because of poor drainage into the bladder, reflux into the ileal segment, and, as a result, excessive electrolyte reabsorption. In the fourth patient, Dr. Burt resolved the problem by bringing the distal end of the ileal ureter, which drained a solitary kidney, to the skin. This resulted in good urinary drainage and prompt stabilization of the patient's condition.

Subsequent to this, in August 1958, a 13-year-old boy was encountered with massive hydroureteronephrosis. The patient presented with hematuria following mild trauma. He underwent Y-V plasty and wedge resection of the bladder neck for primary bladder neck contracture (in retrospect, possibly a valve?) and placement of a suprapubic catheter, but the serum urea nitrogen never fell below 33 mg%. Urinary diversion was performed in September 1958 by Dr. Burt, assisted by Dr. Eliot Leiter. The proximal end of the ileal conduit was passed into the retroperitoneum from the right to left renal pelvis and was anastomosed directly to these structures, allowing excision of the full length of the dilated ureters. The distal end of the conduit was brought to the abdominal wall in the belt line on the right side of the abdomen. The operation, as I recall, lasted about 10 hr, but was attended by a good result.

The technique of pyeloileal cutaneous anastomosis was then refined, and the first ten patients to undergo diversion of this type at Brady were reported by King and Scott in 1962[5]. The operative technique was published in more detail in 1964[7], and may be outlined as follows:

The abdomen is opened through a long midline incision, running from the tip of the xiphoid process to a point midway between the umbilicus and pubis. A paramedian incision, on the side opposite the stoma, is also suitable. After abdominal exploration, the descending colon and spleen are reflected medially, exposing the left kidney. The renal pedicle and pelvis are dissected free, and a length of umbilical tape is passed around the uppermost ureter. The hepatic flexure is then taken down, and the ascending colon is reflected medially, exposing the right kidney. The renal pedicle and pelvis are dissected free, and a length of umbilical tape is passed around the uppermost ureter. After the right pelvis is exposed, a retroperitoneal tunnel, ventral to vena cava and aorta, is constructed between the pelves by gentle blunt and sharp dissection. The peritoneum elevates easily, and the distance to be dsisected is only 4–6 cm. The tunnel is enlarged to the point that it easily accepts the finger (Fig. 3).

This enlargement prevents obstruction of the proximal portion of the conduit, which will be passed through the retroperitoneal tunnel from right to left. A tape is then passed through the tunnel so that it can be relocated easily.

Attention is then turned to preparation of a suitable bowel conduit. Jejunum may be preferable to ileum, since a relatively short mesentery may occasionally prevent the proximal end of an ileal segment from reaching the left kidney without excessive mobilization, which may impair the vascular supply of the segment. The conduit selected must be longer than the average ileal conduit—usually about 25 cm. The blood supply in the mesentery must permit incision to a depth of about 6 cm at either end of the segment to be isolated, leaving the loop supplied by two or more radial arteries. Non-crushing clamps are applied to the bowel to prevent gross peritoneal contamination. The bowel is then divided, between Kocher clamps, at either end of the selected loop. The segment thus isolated is turned superiorly, and bowel continuity is re-established by conventional end-to-end enterostomy. The bowel mesentery is reapproximated with fine silk sutures.

The conduit now lies in the upper abdomen. An opening is made in the retroperitoneum just inferior to the hepatic flexure of the colon. The isolated segment is passed through this into the retroperitoneum, where it comes to rest inferior to the right renal pelvis. Several silk sutures are next placed in the proximal end of the conduit. These are not tied, but are held long. A long curved clamp is used to grasp the tape on the left side of the retroperitoneal tunnel. Using gentle traction on the tape as a guide, the clamp is passed through the tunnel from left to right. The clamp then grasps the sutures in the proximal end of the isolated segment of bowel, which is then gently maneuvered into the retroperitoneal tunnel and across the midline to the left renal pelvis. If the mesentery of the most proximal end of the conduit is constricted, the tunnel may be enlarged inferiorly. If mesenteric length is insufficient, the proximal border may be incised, with care, parallel to the bowel, keeping the artery and vein at the mesenteric border intact. These maneuvers are rarely necessary.

End-to-end left pyeloenterostomy is then performed, using a single layer of 3–0 chromic sutures through all layers of pelvis and bowel. A drain is placed over the anastomoses and exits retroperitoneally through a stab wound in the left flank.

The right kidney is then re-exposed. It is first ascertained that the proximal portion of the conduit lies in the retroperitoneal tunnel without tension. The right renal pelvis or uppermost ureter is then anastomosed to the antimesenteric border of the adjacent portion of the conduit. The incision in the antimesenteric border should be slightly longer than the diameter of

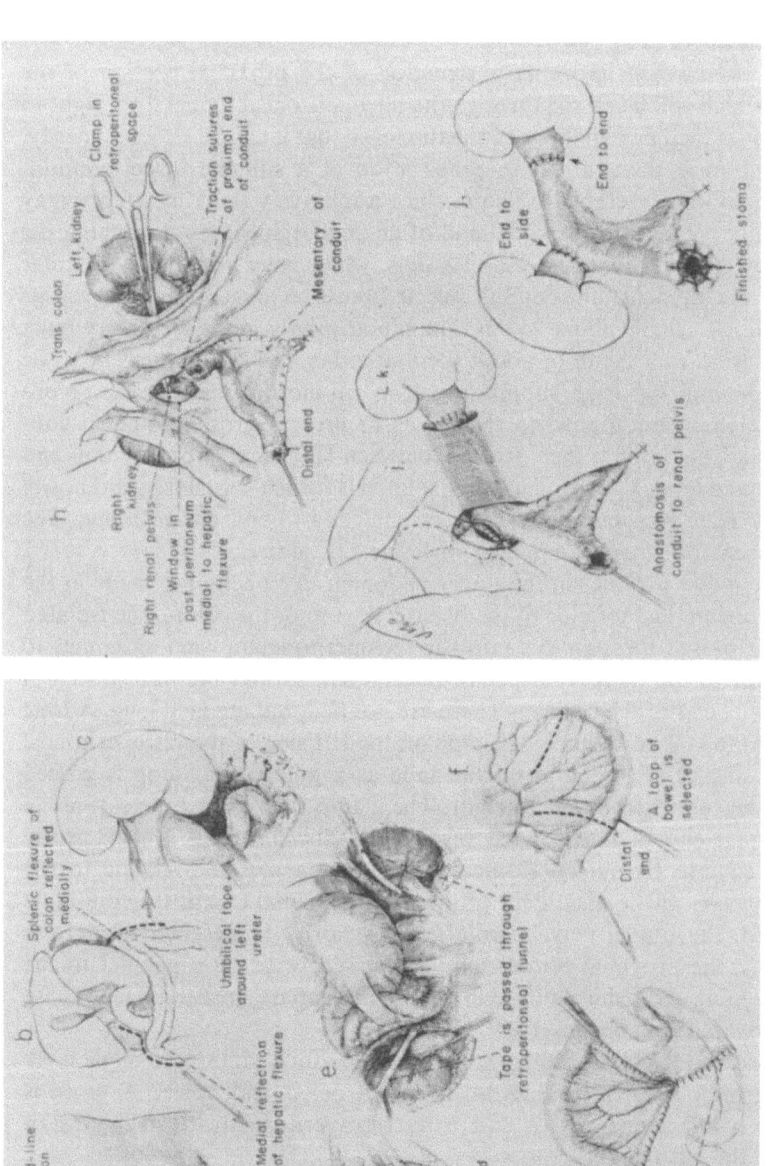

Fig. 3. The technique of pyeloileal cutaneous anastomosis. a: A long midline incision is employed, extending to the xiphoid. b: The isolated loop is high in the abdomen. c: Course of retroperitoneal dissection between the renal pelves. d: The isolated conduit is to be transposed to a position lateral to the ascending colon by drawing it through an opening in the mesentery at the hepatic flexure. e: The conduit is retroperitonealized. The proximal end is led across the midline to the left renal pelvis. Isoperistaltic orientation is maintained. f: The conduit in position. g: The distal end may also exit from the abdomen in a transperitoneal course; however, an extracolonic position is preferred.

the opening in the transected pelvis; otherwise, tissue turned in by the anastomosis tends to narrow the lumen. The anastomoses are checked for leaks.

A site that the conduit will easily reach is next selected for the stoma. This is usually in the belt line to the right of the umbilicus or in the right upper quadrant at least 5 cm below the rib margins. A "cork-bore" plug of abdominal wall, slightly larger than the bowel diameter, is then removed while the edge of the wound is held in normal anatomic position. This prevents the formation of fascial or peritoneal baffles. The distal end of the conduit is led through the stomal opening. Excessive length of conduit is resected, taking care that no tension is placed on the remaining portion. The stoma is then finished in three layers with fine silk sutures—peritoneum and transversalis fascia to serosal surface of bowel, external oblique or anterior rectus fascia to serosa, and skin to serosa to full thickness of the end of the conduit, everting the finished stoma slightly (Fig. 2H).

The high conduit is now entirely in the retroperitoneum. The posterior parietal peritoneum is closed below the hepatic flexure where the mesentery of the conduit passes into the retroperitoneum, preventing a hernia at this site. A drain is usually placed over the site of right pyeloureteral anastomosis and exits in the right flank through a stab wound and posterior to the stoma site. The abdomen is usually closed with retention sutures. This technique was employed in 37 patients reported by Holland et al. in 1968(8).

The majority had marked hydronephrosis prior to surgery (35 of 56 renal units). There were two postoperative deaths, both of patients with pre-existing azotemia. These occurred before dialysis became available, so that surgery in such patients could be done as it is now with preoperative control of uremia. Following high conduit diversion, infection persisted in 40% of these patients because of the marked structural changes, and fixed calyectasis, present in the kidney. Four patients with persistent infection, including two with renal calculi, died with progressive azotemia. In 1968, renal function was deteriorating in two additional patients. These two, and two others operated on after 1967, and not included in Dr. Holland's report, have required dialysis and (renal) transplantation or are awaiting transplantation. In one such patient, diverticula were removed from the hypertrophied bladder, which emptied completely after Y-V plasty, allowing the ureter of the transplanted kidney to be anastomosed to the bladder instead of the ileal conduit. This patient is now well and voiding normally.

In all, 83–85% of patients subjected to pyeloileal cutaneous anastomosis have stabilized or improved, measured in terms of pyelographic appearance and overall kidney function, for periods ranging up to 13 years. More than 50 such operations have now been done at the Brady Institute and at Northwestern University.

One beneficial effect of the generally good results obtained by pyeloileal cutaneous anastomosis has been a renaissance in the use of cutaneous ureterostomy. If the ureterostomy does not function well, the recourse of converting the patient to a "high" conduit at little risk is available. When dilated tortuous ureters are encountered, these may be straightened, brought to the skin in a retroperitoneal course, and implanted into a stoma site prepared as for an ileal conduit, i.e., by excision of a full-thickness plug of the tissues of the abdominal wall, with every expectation of success. When one ureter is near normal in caliber, it can be anastomosed to the dilated mate in the retroperitoneum (transureteroureterostomy) so that both ureters drain across a single stoma. We have recently reported 22 consecutive ureterostomies which were technically successful([9]). When problems are encountered using this technique, it is due to devascularization, occurring when ureters that are excessively convoluted are straightened. This may result in infarction of the distal ureter and consequent stricture. When ureters of normal caliber are brought to the skin, the abdominal wall may compress the small ureter where it passes through the abdominal musculature even though a full-thickness disc has been excised. This often results in edema of the stoma, progressive vascular embarrassment, and consequent necrosis or stricture. When these complications occur, a pyeloileal cutaneous an- astomosis is a reliable operation allowing diversion above the level of ureteral embarrassment. Secondary conduit diversion is most easily performed as soon as it becomes apparent that the ureterostomy is compromised. This can usually be ascertained with certainty within 5–7 days of surgery. Ureteral reaction and fibrosis are worsened when the ureterostomy is intubated prior to re- vision, and this more aggressive approach to revision obviates the necessity for interval nephrostomy drainage. In the past 2 years, two ureterostomy failures of our own, and five similar patients referred from other institutions, have been treated in this manner. The pyeloileal cutaneous anastomosis has worked well in each instance.

The reliability of the conventional ileal conduit, when employed for diversion in patients with ureters of normal or near normal caliber, has also allowed us to employ less reliable procedures as a primary form of diversion. Thus, in recent years, nine children with exstrophy, and normal upper tracts, have been subjected to diversion by ureterosigmoidostomy and are dry without the need to wear an appliance. At this writing, all are doing well, though only two have been followed for longer than 5 years. In one, a trans- ureteroureterostomy is planned to treat slowly progressive right hydroure- teronephrosis.

In summary, the ileal conduit, and its variations, have evolved into an extremely reliable form of urinary diversion. Though 20-year follow-ups are still rare, I can see no reason to suppose that a patient with normal kidneys draining into an established conduit will not have a normal life expectancy, so long as stomal complications are guarded against by periodic examination and calibration.

Technique remains very important to the success of these operations, and great contributions were made at Brady Institute under the guidance of Dr. Scott, whom we honor as a teacher and friend.

REFERENCES

1. Jewett, H. J., King, L. R., and Shelley, W. M. A Study of 365 cases of infiltrating bladder cancer. *J. Urol.* **98**:668–678, 1964.
2. Jewett, H. J. Uretero-intestinal anastomosis in two stages for cancer of the bladder: Modification of original technique and report of 33 cases. *J. Urol.* **52**:536–562, 1944.
3. Cordonnier, J. J. Clinical diversion utilizing an isolated segment of ileum. *J. Urol.* **74**:789–794, 1955.
4. Stamey, T. A., and Scott, W. W. Ureteroileal anastomosis. *Surg. Gynec. Obstet.* **104**:11–24, 1957.
5. King, L. R., and Scott, W. W. Ileal urinary diversion. *J.A.M.A.* **181**:831–839, 1862.
6. Wendel, R. M., and King, L. R. Experimental ablation of ureteral peristalsis. *Invest. Urol.* In Press.
7. King, L. R., and Scott, W. W. Pyeloileocutaneous anastomosis. *Surg. Gynec. Obstet.* **119**:281–292, 1964.
8. Holland, J. M., Schirmer, H. K. M., King, L. R., Gibbons, R. P., and Scott, W. W. Pyeloileal urinary conduit: An 8 year experience in 37 patients. *J. Urol.* **99**:427–433, 1968.
9. Flinn, R. A., King, L. R., McDonald, J. H., and Clark, S. S. Cutaneous ureterostomy: An alternative urinary diversion. *J. Urol.* **105**:358–364, 1971.

Problems in Ileal Conduit Surgery

Joseph D. Schmidt*

Being eligible as a former Brady resident for inclusion in this tribute to Dr. William Wallace Scott is a profound honor in itself. Thus, all the more am I proud to submit the following article to this worthy volume, if only to point out Dr. Scott's significant contributions to the subject of ileal conduit urinary diversion. I cherish my 4 years at Brady—the opportunity to embark on a lifetime of urology and the privilege to be a resident of Dr. William Wallace Scott.

The ileal conduit as a means of supravesical urinary diversion has been widely employed since 1950. The first operations of this nature were performed at The Johns Hopkins Hospital in 1955. All patients at the State University of Iowa Hospitals subjected to ileal diversion from 1961 through 1969 have been reviewed; many of the findings form the basis of this report.

Case records through June 1970 of 178 patients (87 males and 91 females) were studied. Follow-up ranged from 7 days to 105 months. Patients ranged in age at the time of surgery from 16 months to 75 years. Rather than include all statistics gleaned, I have extracted specific problems (Table) 1 which are exemplified by findings in the series.

PATIENT SELECTION

Apart from usual criteria used to evaluate patients, the factor of basic disease process stands out. Two quite different population groups can be

*Associate Professor of Urology, University of Iowa College of Medicine, Iowa City, Iowa.

Table 1. Problems in Ileal Conduit Surgery

1. Patient selection
2. Staging of cystectomy
3. Urine infection
4. Stomal formation
5. Parastomal hernia
6. Conduit length
7. Ureteral transport
8. Ureteral–ileal anastomosis
9. Retroperitonealization
10. Bowel obstruction
11. Radiation changes
12. Wound closure
13. Additional procedures
14. Experience of surgeon

distinguished—those with underlying benign disease and those with underlying malignancy. Patients with benign disease were younger at the time of surgery (average age of 13.7 years) than those with malignancy (average age 50.6 years). No patient aged 70 or older survived more than 7 months regardless of disease.

Morbidity and mortality were disparate between the two groups (Table 2). Early and late mortality were similar in the benign group, whereas early mortality was greater in the malignant group. The late mortality rate was high (50%) for the malignant group, probably stemming from the natural history of the underlying cancer as well as the higher complication rate seen in such patients. At the University of Iowa Hospitals no patient in the benign category has died in the early postoperative period (0–30 days) since 1963. Only one patient in the benign group has died in the late postoperative period (after 30 days) in the last 7 years. The causes of death are listed in Table 3.

The pattern of complications, major and minor, is listed in Table 4. Note that early postoperative complications were more common in the malignant group, whereas later the reverse was true. I believe this occurs because of deaths from carcinomatosis, while the longer survival of the patients in the benign group allows them time to develop more complications such as acute pyelonephritis, stomal stenosis, peristomal dermatitis, stomal irritation, urinary calculi, acidosis, pyocystis, and ureteral–ileal obstruction.

Table 2. Mortality Related to Ileal Diversion

Disease	Early		Late		Total	
Benign	3/130	(2.3%)	3/130	(2.3%)	6/130	(4.6%)
Malignant	3/48	(6.2%)	24/48	(50%)	27/48	(56%)
All patients	6/178	(3.4%)	27/178	(15%)	33/178	(18%)

Table 3. Causes of Death in Ileal Diversion Patients

Malignant disease (27)	
Carcinomatosis	22
Sepsis	3
Pulmonary embolism	1
Uremia	1
Benign disease (6)	
Sepsis	4
Tuberculosis	1
Unknown	1

Table 4. Complications of Ileal Conduit Diversion

Complication	No. of patients	Incidence (%)
Early		
Benign	36/130	28
Malignant	24/48	50
Late		
Benign	108/127	85
Malignant	20/45	44

Ninety separate hospitalizations were required for nonsurgical treatment of complications. That considerable additional surgery is generated by the ileal conduit operation is documented by the need for 113 secondary surgical procedures. Included were stomal revisions (27), ureteral–ileal anastomosis revisions (15), lysis of adhesions for bowel obstruction (11), and removal of urinary calculi (nine).

STAGING OF CYSTECTOMY

Surprisingly, cystectomy was required in only seven of 130 patients (5%) with benign disease. Each cystectomy, indicated for recurrent or persistent pyocystis, was performed as a separate operation rather than in combination with diversion.

Twenty-seven of 48 patients (56%) with malignant disease underwent cystectomy: at the time of diversion in nine, with exenteration and diversion in 11, and as a staged procedure, e.g., bladder carcinoma, in seven.

Cystectomy was *not* indicated or performed in 144 patients (81%).

URINE INFECTION

Reviews of ileal diversions describe a variable incidence of positive urine cultures or clinical infections such as acute pyelonephritis. In this series of those tested preoperatively, 15% had sterile urine while 85% had infection. Of those cultured at some time in the postoperative period, only

3 % had sterile urine while 97 % were infected. Of those having sterile urine before diversion, urine infection occurred postoperatively in all tested. Of those infected before diversion, 98 % remained infected.

Should more vigorous therapy of preoperative infection be carried out in an attempt to sterilize the urine at the time of diversion? What is the significance of a positive culture from ileal conduit urine in an asymptomatic patient? Is there a "normal flora of pathogens" in such urine because of the ileal milieu? And, if such a culture is significant, should we be more vigorous in its treatment? One approach to these questions is a careful bacteriological study of ileal conduits and their contained urine.

STOMAL FORMATION

Many of the early and late problems focused on the stoma, e.g., stomal stenosis with subsequent high conduit residuals or hydroureteronephrosis. Obstruction has occurred at three levels: skin, fascia, and muscle.

My method of stomal formation includes preoperative examination of the patient's abdomen to determine optimal position. I recommend removal of a full-thickness cylinder of abdominal wall to avoid any "shutter" effect by muscle or obstruction by fascia or skin. Such a core can be taken to the posterior fascia at the onset and completed through the peritoneum later. If stomal position is undecided, the full thickness of abdominal wall can be removed after much of the conduit surgery has been completed. I prefer to fashion the stomal channel prior to the distortion that occurs after the peritoneal cavity has been entered. A circular incision adequate for the patient's ileum does not predispose to stenosis.

PARASTOMAL HERNIA

Parastomal hernia occurred in five patients early in the postoperative period—from the third through seventh days—associated with ileus, abdominal distention, and bowel obstruction. The clinical clues included a serous ooze (really peritoneal fluid) from the lateral margin of the ileal stoma, and, on removal of skin sutures, a knuckle of small bowel presented. Treatment consisted of immediate open reduction of the hernia with suturing of the defect from within the peritoneal cavity and from the stomal side. Parastomal hernia occurred in the late postoperative period in three patients, in one of whom a Richter's type hernia was noted.

Such a complication can be prevented by suturing of the conduit in three layers or tiers as it traverses the abdominal wall. Firstly, a layer of interrupted 0000 or 000 silk between the peritoneum–posterior fascial layer and seromuscular layer of the conduit; secondly, and most importantly, a layer of interrupted 00 or 0 silk between the anterior rectus fascia and conduit seromuscular layer; and, thirdly, a layer of interrupted 0000 or 00000 sutures, absorbable or nonabsorbable, between the skin and full thickness of the conduit stoma (Fig. 1 and 2).

All sutures can be placed from the outside, although some of the peritoneal layer can be placed from within the abdomen. The greatest attention must be taken, especially at the anterior fascial level, to place sutures close enough to each other and to the mesenteric insertion to avoid both defects for herniation and embarrassment of blood supply.

I prefer to perform this portion of the surgery immediately after closure and fixation of the proximal conduit. In this way, the conduit is well fixed

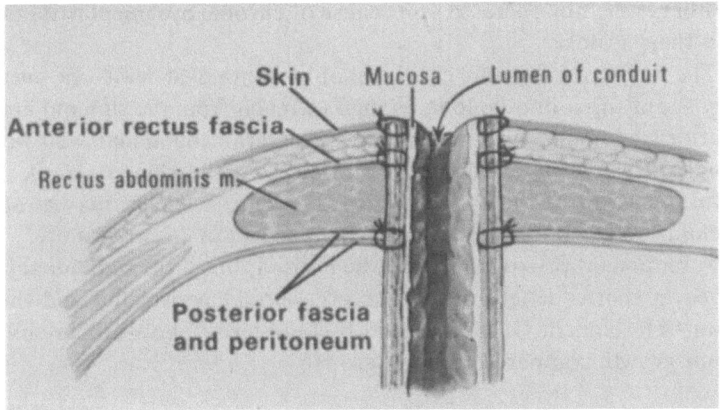

Fig. 1. Cross-section of ileal conduit traversing abdominal wall defect. Note three-layer fixation.

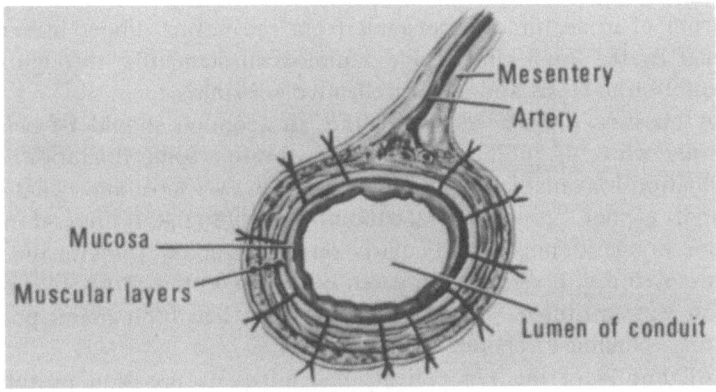

Fig. 2. Coronal section of ileal conduit demonstrating placement of sutures with reference to mesentery. View at level of anterior fascia.

at each end making the ureteral–ileal anastomoses relatively simple to perform.

CONDUIT LENGTH

That long conduits with increased mucosal surface for urine absorption increase the possibility of hyperchloremic acidosis is well documented. Even an adequate length of conduit can lead to hyperchloremic acidosis in the presence of distal obstruction. In this series a late metabolic acidosis, often with hyperchloremia, occurred in 16 patients (9%). Shortening of the conduit was performed in two patients, with improvement in renal function. The others were not operated on because of chronic pyelonephritis contributing to their acidosis.

The segment of ileum chosen should contain at least one mesenteric artery supplying it and be long enough to reach from the sigmoid across the posterior abdominal wall and along the lateral abdominal wall or cecum through the anterior abdominal wall defect to the skin. A sterile ruler is helpful in measuring the length needed. Fifteen centimeters may be adequate in a child, while a large adult may need a conduit of 25 cm or more.

A redundant proximal end can be excised, but if the redundancy is generalized, a shorter length of small bowel should be isolated and the entire conduit refashioned. Of interest will be long-term follow-ups in children of conduit growth compared to body growth.

URETERAL TRANSPORT

The conduit, if of proper length, isoperistaltic and unobstructed, quickly transports urine to the stoma. But if transport from the calyces through the ureteral termini is deficient, the operation will fall short of its goal. The spectrum of urine transport extends from the normal upper urinary tract (normal by the usual clinical and radiological standards) through degrees of dilatation to stasis and lack of effective peristalsis.

A question often asked is whether the conduit should be performed electively when the ureters are normal or after some dilatation occurs? Information is available to support either view, yet most agree that if urine transport is poor, "routine" ileal conduit is likely to fail. If ureteral transport is poor or questionable, particularly on cine studies, I advise the "high" ileal or pyeloileal diversion. On seven occasions in this series, pyeloileal diversion was instituted. Two of these patients had been doing poorly on "routine" conduit diversion.

All but 14 of the 178 patients had adequate pre- and postoperative pyelograms. Comparisons (Table 5) show that a significant proportion of patients with initially normal upper tracts did later undergo deterioration.

Table 5. Excretory Urographic Status in Ileal Conduit Diversion

Normal preop study (58)		
Postop: Normal	40	(69%)
Deteriorated	18	(31%)
Abnormal preop study (106)		
Postop: Normal	30⎫	(71%)
Improved	45⎭	
Unchanged	19	(18%)
Deteriorated	12	(11%)
No postop study beyond 10 days	14	

Yet up to 71 % of those patients with abnormal upper tracts preoperatively did show improvement later, even to normality.

That abnormal upper tracts undergo further deterioration can be considered as natural history of the underlying disease. But deterioration of any upper tract also can be due to technical errors resulting in ureteral–ileal or conduit obstruction with subsequent ureteral involvement.

URETERAL–ILEAL ANASTOMOSIS

A satisfactory anastomosis results when full thickness of ureter, spatulated if needed, is sutured to full thickness of ileum at its antimesenteric or posterior surface. To avoid obstruction, a small piece of mucosa should be removed at the time of ileotomy. Fine chromic catgut interrupted sutures, 0000 or 00000, are placed starting with the apex and alternating each lateral border until a watertight anastomosis is completed. Helpful here is a grooved director in placing sutures within the bowel and ureteral lumina. All knots are on the outside. One or two fixation sutures between the posterior wall of the conduit and the anterior wall of the ureter are helpful in localizing the anastomosis as well as aiding in its stability.

The left ureter should be deviated as little as possible from its normal course. The left ureteral–ileal anastomosis can be made on either the medial or lateral side of the mesosigmoid. It is preferable to bring the conduit to the left ureter through the mesosigmoid rather than bring the left ureter to the conduit.

Each anastomosis should be tested by gentle instillation of sterile saline by bulb syringe at the stoma. As the conduit fills, leaks can be detected and repaired by additional sutures under direct vision. Although some reflux is bound to occur, no postoperative problems attributable to this maneuver have resulted.

A second reinforcing layer of sutures is not needed. Approximately one half of the operations in this series were performed with a two-layer ureteral–ileal anastomosis. No significant differences in results were noted. Splinting catheters, used in 35 of 178 cases, are optional and, if the anastomoses are watertight, are not indicated.

No attempt was made to create an antireflux anastomosis, yet on follow-up ileograms and intravenous pyelograms, nine patients (with 12 ureteral–ileal anastomoses) demonstrated neither reflux nor obstruction. A safe, reproducible antireflux method for ureteral–ileal anastomoses would be a valuable addition to the procedure.

RETROPERITONEALIZATION

Attempts to retroperitonealize the conduit vary from none to complete displacement posterior to the parietal peritoneum. My technique utilizes the flaps of posterior parietal peritoneum elevated for ureteral dissection. Suturing of these flaps to the seromuscular portion of the conduit around each ureteral–ileal anastomosis places these junctions retroperitoneal (Fig. 3, 4, and 5). Should surgery be required later here, a retroperitoneal approach can be utilized. Also, prophylactic or therapeutic drainage of urine leakage can be handled completely retroperitoneally. The proximal conduit can be retroperitonealized via such a maneuver in the area of the mesosigmoid.

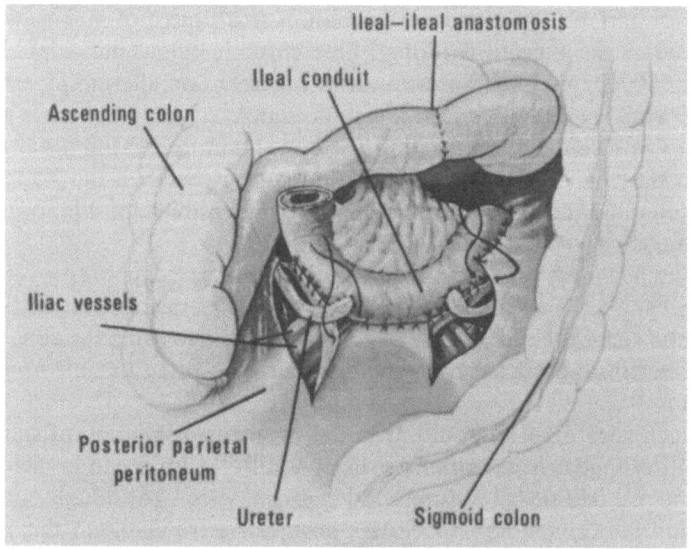

Fig. 3. Retroperitonealization of ureteral–ileal anastomoses utilizing paraureteral flaps of posterior parietal peritoneum.

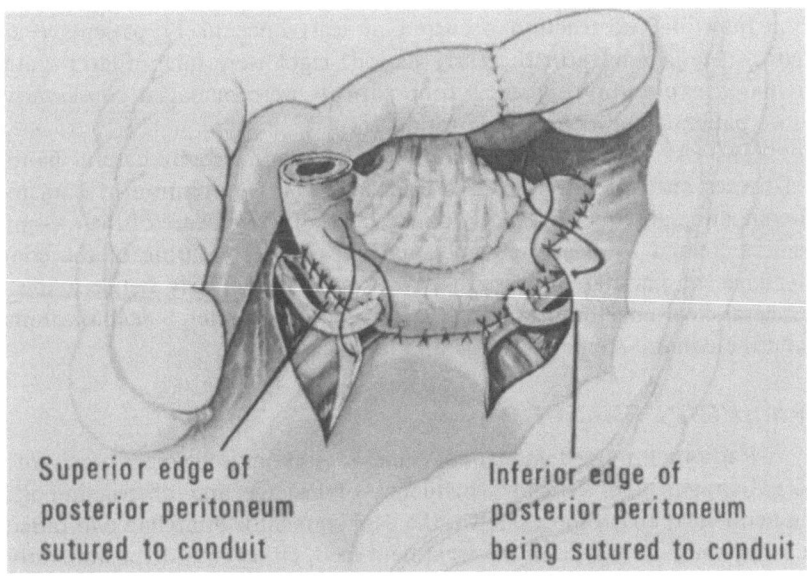

Fig. 4. Closeup of retroperitonealization procedure.

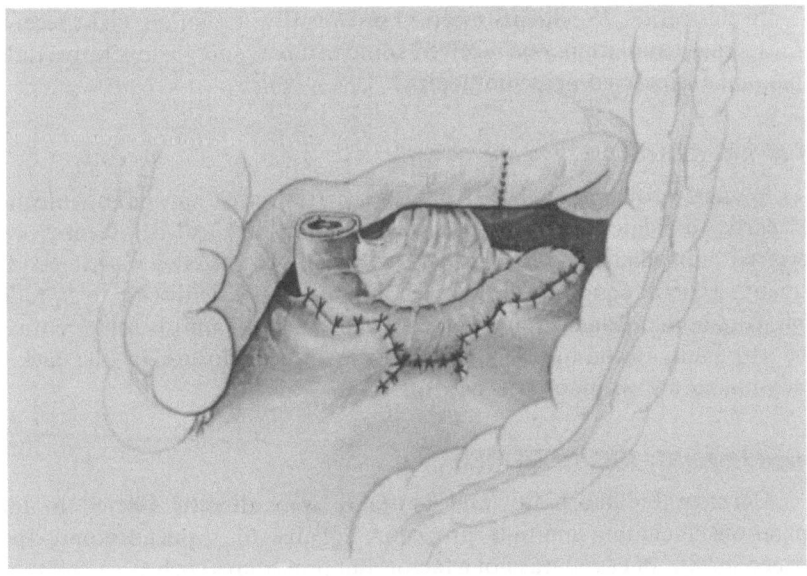

Fig. 5. Retroperitonealization completed.

BOWEL OBSTRUCTION

Intestinal obstruction occurred at least once in 17 patients (9.6%). Nine instances were in the early period; eight were later. Eleven patients required exploration, whereas four patients were managed conservatively. Two patients died before exploration.

The risk of bowel obstruction can be minimized by careful handling of tissues and special care to certain details: (a) prevention of parastomal hernia and subsequent obstruction (see above); (b) closure of the mesenteric defect created by ileal segment isolation; and (c) suturing of the conduit to adjacent parietal or visceral peritoneum, particularly between the two ureteral–ileal anastomoses and between the right ureteral–ileal anastomosis and the conduit's entry into the abdominal wall.

RADIATION CHANGES

Radiotherapy for malignancy may result in ischemic fibrosis of the distal ureters and a greater incidence of leakage and obstruction at the ureteral–ileal anastomoses. Also, the ileal segment is more liable to radiation change since it may lie in the treatment field, either pre- or postoperatively. The ureter proximal to the radiation field can be utilized to avoid this complication. Some advocate using the transverse colon as a conduit, ensuring that the anastomoses and the conduit are well away from the radiation field.

In this series, 25 patients received preoperative radiation, eight received postoperative radiation, one received combined pre- and postoperative radiation, and 14 received no radiotherapy.

WOUND CLOSURE

Wound problems included dehiscence (six early, one late), infection (11 early, four late), and incisional hernia (four late). All dehiscences were repaired immediately, whereas hernia repair was elective based on the patient's general condition. Etiologies included (a) basic disease, e.g., radiation, carcinoma, urinary infection, azotemia, obesity, and the older patient; and (b) faulty technique, e.g., inadequate fascial closure or the lack of retention sutures in poor-risk patients.

ADDITIONAL PROCEDURES

Considerable morbidity and mortality were directly related to long operations including multiple procedures (Table 6). Appendectomy (performed in 78% of cases) was not a factor. But procedures such as gastrostomy, anterior exenteration, small bowel resection, and hysterectomy were signifi-

Table 6. Additional Procedures Performed with Ileal Diversion

Gastrostomy	6	Orchiopexy	2
Anterior exenteration	6	Nephrectomy, ureterectomy	2
Nephrostomy	4	Meckel's diverticulectomy	2
Orchiectomy	3	Hysterectomy	2
Partial bladder resection	3	Sigmoid colostomy	1
Small bowel resection	3	Cystolithotomy	1
Salpingo-oophorectomy	3		

cant. Gastrostomy is no better than nasogastric tube drainage and should be avoided. Staging procedures to minimize postoperative complications is a better alternative.

EXPERIENCE OF SURGEON

Approximately 75 % of the patients were operated on and cared for by the resident staff with attending staff supervision. Patients with meningomyelocele (74), usually falling into a category of state financial support, were with few exceptions operated on by chief residents. In a university urology residency training program, major surgery such as the ileal conduit and treatment of its complications must necessarily be handled by the resident with adequate staff supervision. The majority of such operations are performed in university medical centers and must continue to be utilized to train residents, many of whom remain in a similar environment.

SUMMARY

Using information gleaned from 178 patients undergoing ileal conduit urinary diversion, 14 specific problems have been described. Recommendations to solve these problems and improve overall results have been made. The ileal conduit diversion remains a major operative procedure dealt with most often in the university medical center, where it serves as a significant portion of the training of the urology resident.

REFERENCES

1. Bricker, E. M. Bladder substitution after pelvic evisceration. *Surg. Clin. N. Am.* **30**;1511, 1950.
2. Burnham, J. P., and Farrer, J. A group experience with uretero-ileal-cutaneous anastomosis for urinary diversion: Results and complications of the isolated ileal conduit (Bricker procedure) in 96 patients. *J. Urol.* **83**:622, 1960.
3. Campbell, W. A., and Buchtel, H. A. Advantages of high ileac conduit. *J. Urol.* **91**:66, 1964.
4. Cohen, S. M., and Persky, L. A ten-year experience with ureteroileostomy. *Arch. Surg.* **95**:278, 1967.

5. Cordonnier, J. J. Clinical diversion utilizing an isolated segment of ileum. *J. Urol.* **74**:789, 1955.

6. Cordonnier, J. J. Ileal bladder substitution: An analysis of 78 cases. *J. Urol.* **77**:714, 1957

7. Creevy, C. D. Renal complications after ileac diversion of the urine in non-neoplastic disorders. *J. Urol.* **83**:394, 1960.

8. Holland, J. M., Schirmer, H. K. A., King, L. R., Gibbons, R. P., and Scott, W. W. Pyelo-ileal urinary conduit: An 8-year experience in 37 patients. *J. Urol.* **99**:427, 1968.

9. Jaffe, B. M., Bricker, E. M., and Butcher, H. R., Jr. Surgical complications of ileal segment urinary diversion. *Ann. Surg.* **167**:367, 1968.

10. Kafetsioulis, A., and Swinney, J. Urinary diversion by ileal conduit. A long-term follow-up. *Brit. J. Urol.* **40**:1, 1968.

11. King, L. R., and Scott, W. W. Ileal urinary diversion. Success of pyeloileocutaneous anastomosis in correction of hydroureteroneophrosis persisting after ureteroileocutaneous anastomosis. *J.A.M.A.* **181**:831, 1962.

12. King, L. R., and Scott, W. W. Pyeloileocutaneous anastomosis. *Surg. Gynec. Obstet.* **119**:281, 1964.

13. Scott, W. W. Methods of urinary diversion in radical pelvic surgery. *Clin. Obstet. Gynec.* **8**:726, 1965.

14. Stamey, T. A., and Scott, W. W. Ureteral ileal anastomosis. *Surg. Gynec. Obstet.* **104**:11, 1957.

15. Sunshine, H., Cordonnier, J. J., and Butcher, H. Bilateral pyeloileostomy. *J. Urol.* **92**:358, 1964.

Renal Failure—Remarks On Its Causes

David M. Davis*

For at least 150 years urologists have known that obstruction to the outflow of urine from the urinary tract increases its susceptibility to infection with pyogenic microorganisms. As long as the obstruction persists, infection is more difficult to eradicate. Elimination of the obstruction often leads to spontaneous disappearance of the infection.

Many nonurological physicians are unwilling to accept the dicta stated in the preceding paragraph unless the obstruction is gross and unmistakable even if no special diagnostic methods have been used. For them, the chief reliance in the treatment of urinary tract infections is upon the use of antibiotic drugs, and they content themselves with the statement that there is "no demonstrable obstruction."

This difference of opinion can be resolved only by a precise definition of "obstruction," so that there can never be any doubt as to whether obstruction is present or not.

Considering the means of propulsion of the urine from the pelvis to the exterior of the body—that is, peristalsis in the ureters, periodic voiding of the bladder and urethra—one can justifiably postulate that an obstructive lesion is one that prevents the passage of urine through the urinary passages at normal pressures and normal rates of flow. Until quite recently, we did not know what these normal pressures and rates of flow are, so that we could not be certain about the existence of minor degrees of obstruction.

At the present time, we can measure intravesical and intraurethral pressures and voiding flow rates with comparative ease and a high degree of

*Professor of Urology, Emeritus, Thomas Jefferson University School of Medicine, Philadelphia, Pennsylvania.

accuracy. Fredrik Kiil showed how intrapelvic and intraureteral pressures—including the contraction and resting pressures of peristaltic waves—could be measured accurately by simple and safe procedures. It can therefore now be stated that urine should normally be propelled through the ureters at contraction pressures of 20–24 cm of water, that the resting pressures between contractions should not be over 4 cm of water, unless intraperitoneal pressure, which affects intraureteral resting pressure, is raised as by straining, and that voiding should occur at a flow rate of at least 22 ml/sec (in the adult) with bladder pressure of not over 40 mm of mercury. From observations already made, we know that intraureteral pressures can rise abnormally high before any ureterectasis is demonstrable and that the voiding rate can be normal even through an obstructed urethra, thanks to an elevated intravesical pressure due to muscular hypertrophy of the detrusor.

These procedures have not as yet come into general use. If and when they do, many slight and moderate obstructions, formerly ignored, will be disclosed and subjected to correction. I have little doubt that this will appreciably improve that treatment of chronic and recurrent urinary tract infections.

This in itself is a very desirable objective, but upon careful thought, other important possibilities appear. If it is indeed true that many slight and moderate obstructions go unrecognized, and do help to maintain chronic and recurrent infection, may it not be that such combinations of obstruction and infection play a significant role in the causation of renal failure? In an effort to gain knowledge concerning this hypothesis, I have attended, over a period of 3 or 4 years, the clinics of the Nephrology Department at the Jefferson Hospital (now the Hospital of the Thomas Jefferson University). From this experience I gather very definite impressions. First, the urological history—or anamnesis, as the late Dr. Barker would say—is usually very inadequately taken and recorded. Second, the presence or absence of urinary tract infection is often inadequately explored, and very inadequately followed during the period in which the patient is under observation. Third, the provision for competent and interested urological evaluation of all cases is often inadequate, and too often the decision as to the necessity and extent of urological examinations is made not by a urologist but by the nephrology staff.

It must be said that these omissions are understandable in the light of the onerous responsibilities the nephrologists have of saving and supporting the unfortunate patients whose kidneys are already irreparably damaged. Nevertheless, the urologist, equipped with his new and exciting modalities for accurate and complete diagnosis, can be of the utmost value to them in the effort to unravel the etiological puzzle of renal failure. This effort, of course—which, if successful, may lead to effective preventive measures—

is an inescapable obligation of everyone dealing with renal failure—including, besides nephrologists and urologists, the larger groups of pediatricians, internists, and general practitioners.

At present, renal failure is usually ascribed to pyelonephritis, glomerulonephritis, arteriosclerosis, or lupus. Biopsies, especially needle biopsies, are relied upon heavily in making the distinction among these entities. There is much disagreement among pathologists, as well as among clinicians, as to the dependability of diagnoses so made. Experienced observers such as Paul Kimmelstiel state that chronic pyelonephritis and glomerulonephritis can easily be confused. In addition, one must consider the possibility of pictures which may further confuse the issue, due to coexistent arteriosclerosis, virus infection, allergic changes, toxic chemicals, amyloidosis, lupus, or "burned-out" bacterial infections. In other words, kidney biopsy in a patient already in renal failure either tells us little or may deceive us as to the underlying primary cause of the trouble.

There is only one answer to this problem. Renal failure may be referred to as a slowly developing, chronic disease with which, in all too many cases, we are familiar only in its terminal stages. To link up all the stages and form a clear concept of the origin and progress of the disease will demand the understanding and cooperation of the other medical disciplines already mentioned. Pediatricians, even if they feel that an individual patient showing some evidence of urinary tract disease does not need thorough examination and radical treatment, should endeavor to pass the patient along, with his record, to an understanding general practitioner of internist who will keep watch to assure that the condition does not grow worse in later life, or even continue for too long a time.

All physicians, in cases where symptoms persist or where long-continued or repeated courses of antibiotics are felt necessary, should insist that thorough examination be carried out long before uremia begins, to discover definitely whether some form of preventive treatment is possible. Only in this way can we learn the natural history of renal failure and be able to devise rational and effective means of prevention.

Renin and Erythropoietin Levels in Uremic and Anephric Man*

Gerald P. Murphy† and Edwin A. Mirand†

The association of uremic renal disease with hypertension and anemia has been clinically identifiable for some time. The kidney is known to play a significant role in the production or release, or both, of two substances: erythropoietin (ESF), a hormone active in regulating the production of red blood cells[1], and renal renin[2]. Levels of both of these hormones, ESF and renal renin, may be altered significantly in the presence of uremic renal insufficiency[2-4].

Thus, the uremic and renoprival state in man presented an opportunity for the study of the presence and interrelationships of renin and ESF under these conditions. The presence of these hormones was studied in anephric patients maintained on intermittent hemodialysis prior to renal allotransplantation.

MATERIALS AND METHODS

This study included 23 male and 22 female patients, 14–64 years of age, whose clinical conditions had previously been diagnosed as chronic renal failure (Table 1). When possible, patients were studied first with untreated uremic renal failrue (blood urea nitrogen greater than 140 mg%) and then periodically. Thus patients were observed at admission, on biweekly hem-

*This study was supported in part by USPHS Grant CA-07745 and the J. A. Hartford Foundation, Inc.
†Roswell Park Memorial Institute (New York State Department of Health) and State University of New York at Buffalo, Buffalo, New York.

Table 1. Causes of Renal Failure in Patients Studied

Pyelonephritis	18
Glomerulonephritis	15
Nephrosclerosis	5
Polycystic disease	5
Other (congenital, familial)	2
Total	45

odialysis, and after bilateral nephrectomy. No patient was under pharmacological therapy at the time of collection of blood specimens. The anephric period varied for each patient. During the observation period, all patients were maintained on a diet containing 40 g of protein and 0.5 g of salt, with variable fluid intake determined chiefly by the presence or absence of kidneys. Patients were classified as hypertensive when the diastolic blood pressure was greater than 100 mm Hg on three successive determinations while on bed rest in the hospital[2]. Although numerous clinical and biochemical determinations were performed, the present report deals only with ESF, renin, serum sodium, hematocrit, and blood urea nitrogen levels in patients with renal insufficiency.

Periodically, samples of venous blood were aseptically obtained and stored at $2-0$ C for later assay. This method of short storage does not abolish or diminish ESF activity[3,4]. When patients were treated with hemodialysis, samples were collected on the day before hemodialysis.

Samples were thawed and later subcutaneously injected into polycythemic Ha/ICR Swiss mice. At least five polycythemic mice were employed to assay each pooled test specimen. Each mouse received 0.1 ml of test fluid for 4 successive days. On the fifth day, 1 μc of radioactive iron (Fe^{59}) in the form of ferrous sulfate was intravenously injected into the tail vein. Animals were killed and bled from the dorsal aorta 24 hr later. The percentage uptake of Fe^{59} in 24 hr was a measure of the ESF level. Assay animals with hematocrit readings less than 60% at the end of this period were not used. This method precludes release of endogenous ESF by test mice.

Erythropoietin values are expressed both as percentage uptake of Fe^{59} in 24 hr and as the following ratio:

$$\frac{\text{24-hr percentage } Fe^{59} \text{ uptake with test plasma}}{\text{24-hr percentage } Fe^{59} \text{ uptake with saline control}}$$

This ratio normally ranges between 1.0 and 1.3 in intact man and animals.

Renin (ng %) in stored plasma specimens was assayed by the method of Gunnells[5]. This method of bioassay differs from radioimmunoassay in that substances other than renin can give "renin-like" assay responses. This is especially important in the anephric state where radioimmunoassay results are generally low or absent.

RESULTS

Uremic Man

Table 2 shows the levels of plasma renin, ESF, ESF ratio, hematocrit (Hct), blood urea nitrogen (BUN), and serum sodium in uremic patients kept on maintenance hemodialysis. These data are based on more than 106 observations of all patients prior to bilateral nephrectomy.

Higher levels of renin were present in hypertensive uremic patients than in normotensive patients ($p < 0.01$). No significant difference between hypertensive and normotensive uremic patients was observed in level of serum sodium, Hct, or BUN (Table 2). Significant levels of ESF and ESF ratio were noted, but these levels were similar in normotensive and hypertensive uremic patients. With a Hct level in the range of 20–21%, however, a higher level of plasma ESF would have been expected. For ten nonuremic normotensive patients with hematocrits in the range of 20–21%, plasma ESF levels averaged $8.2 \pm 0.6\%$ 24-hr uptake. It appears that the uremic state,

Table 2. Plasma Renin and Erythropoietin (ESF) Levels in Uremic Patients with Renal Insufficiency[a]

Period	Plasma renin (ng %)	Plasma ESF (24-hr Fe^{59} uptake)	ESF ratio	Hct (vol %)	BUN (mg %)	Serum sodium (meq/liter)
Normotensive (19 patients)	874.7 ±130.9	2.50 ±1.20	5.6 +2.6	21.6 ±0.5	86.9 ±5.1	132.5 ±1.5
Hypertensive (26 patients)	1572.2 ±128	2.18 ±0.81	5.03 ±1.98	20.97 ±0.6	84.1 ±6.4	132.7 ±0.82

[a] All values are mean $\pm$ 1 SE. One hundred and six observations were made in each group. Normal range for plasma renin in our laboratory is 400–600 ng %. Normal level of plasma ESF is 0.38% 24-hr Fe^{59} uptake in patients with a normal hematocrit.

Table 3. Plasma Renin Response to Dialysis in Renal Insufficiency[a]

Condition	No. of patients	Plasma renin (ng %)
Prior to treatment	21	1070.8 ±171.5
Following prolonged (30 days) treatment	24	1429.3 ±207

[a] Normal range for plasma renin in our laboratory is 400–600 ng %. All values are mean $\pm$ 1 SE.

regardless of whether a patient is normotensive or hypertensive, affects the level of plasma ESF.

Table 3 summarizes renin levels in several patients studied initially and after institution of maintenance of hemodialysis and dietary control. Dietary regulation, including successful sodium restriction, as well as maintenance of hemodialysis, did not result in lowering of peripheral renin in either normotensive or hypertensive patients (Table 4). Among normotensive patients, however, it was the patients initially hypertensive or hypertensive following dialysis who still had higher levels of renin.

Anephric Man

Observations were made on anephric patients. The periods of the renoprival state varied from 7 to 154 days. The duration of the anephric state was in the main variably influenced by the availability of a suitable living or cadaveric donor kidney. Levels of BUN and Hct were relatively constant (Table 5). The data shown in Table 5 confirm previous observations that extrarenal renin, or renin-like substances as well as extrarenal ESF[3,4], are present in anephric man. Extrarenal ESF levels were present in the plasma to a detectable and significant degree during all periods of the anephric state. It interesting to note that the highest levels of ESF in the present study were not present at the same times as when high levels of renin-like substances were observed. Such observations suggest an active conversion to active pressor substance during these periods, and not a uremic backlog or metabolic pile-up. These results with the bioassay technique are different from radioimmunoassay[5]. The significance of this is under current study.

Some patients remained hypertensive despite the anephric state (Table 6). Comparison of such hypertensive anephric patients with normotensive

Table 4. Plasma Renin Response to Dialysis in Patients
with Renal Insufficiency[a]

Condition	No. of patients	Plasma renin (ng %)
Normotensive on initial dialysis	3	677 ±85
Normotensive after dialysis (30 days)	7	837.3 ±285
Hypertensive on initial dialysis	10	1096.4 ±251
Hypertension sustained after dialysis (30 days)	21	1557.5 ±295

[a] All values are mean ± 1 SE.

Table 5. Plasma Renin and Erythropoietin (ESF) Levels in Anephric Man[a]

Days anephric	No. of patients	Plasma renin (ng %)	Plasma ESF (24-hr Fe^{59} uptake)	ESF ratio	Hct (vol %)	BUN (mg %)
0–7	23	972.8 ±167	1.67 ±0.44	4.23 ±1.06	22.3 ±0.90	77.5 ±7.6
8–14	22	893.05 ±160	1.23 ±0.18	2.91 ±0.94	21.7 ±0.95	75.2 ±7.1
15–28	20	821.3 ±152	2.71 ±1.32	6.28 ±3.67	21.2 ±0.54	66.7 ±4.7
29–42	17	925.2 ±227	1.41 ±0.54	4.86 ±1.86	21.31 ±0.85	70 ±6.0
43–70	5	1359.2 ±218	1.13 ±0.22	3.65 ±0.60	21.0 ±0.55	86 ±4.0
71–98	4	1247.3 ±396.3	1.06 ±0.13	1.81 ±0.70	18.0 ±0.20	76 ±5.1
99–126	2	1493.4 ±441	1.17 ±0.33	2.72 ±0.60	21.0 ±0.7	53 ±4.2
127–154	1	658 ±211	2.74 ±0.83	6.54 ±0.21	19.0 ±0.6	82 ±7.6

[a] All values are mean ± 1 SE.

Table 6. Plasma Renin Levels in Anephric Man[a]

Days anephric	Plasma renin (ng %)	
	Normotensive	Hypertensive
0–7	520.4 ±81.6	959.2 ±133
8–14	1080.7 ±371	598.4 ±90.4
15–28	1153.5 ±571	695.6 ±74.8

[a] All values are mean ± 1 SE.

anephric patients failed to demonstrate higher levels of renin in hypertensive patients, particularly after 7 days. In fact, higher levels of renin were observed in the normotensive anephric patients after 7 days (Table 6). All anephric patients were hospitalized and on rigid control of fluid and dietary salt. Differences in salt and water intake are thus not the apparent cause for the sustained hypertension in anephric man. Other mechanisms not involving the renin–renin substrate system must be operative.

DISCUSSION

The present investigation reaffirms our original observations that an extrarenal source for ESF exists in man[3,4]. It is unlikely that any blood transfusion or pre-existing renal insufficiency may account for these levels of extrarenal ESF, since the measured half-life of ESF in the plasma has been noted to be only a few hours[6]. Similarly, significant levels of ESF were detected in normotensive or hypertensive uremic patients with renal insufficiency (Table 2), although patients without renal insufficiency but with hematocrit levels in the same range exhibited higher levels of ESF, indicating that the uremic state does in some way interfere with ESF production or release, or both. It was also noted that hypertension in the presence (Table 2) or absence (Tables 5 and 6) of kidneys in these uremic states was not associated with higher levels of ESF.

Renal ischemia can affect renal ESF production or release, but what factors influence extrarenal ESF production or release are not known. It has been postulated that an inhibitor substance from diseased kidneys may prevent normal erythropoietin production or release and thus interfere with erythropoietic responses that contribute to anemia in the uremic state[7]. It is also felt that hemodialysis and nephrectomy may alter this inhibitor substance to an unknown degree. If this should be the case, it could perhaps affect extrarenal ESF in man, since extrarenal ESF varies sharply on a day-to-day basis in anephric man, as is demonstrated by our present and past observations[8].

If renin is causally related to uremic hypertension, then it should be anticipated that uremic hypertensive patients with elevated plasma renin levels would be helped by nephrectomy. Similar conclusions have been reached by others[9-13]. Even so, we have observed normotensive anephric patients with elevated plasma renin or renin-like substances (Table 6). Accordingly, it cannot be said that renin is causally related to hypertension in all cases of uremic hypertension. Besides, as Table 6 shows, some patients can remain hypertensive in the anephric state without developing elevated levels of renin.

It thus appears that other mechanisms must be evoked in these instances. We have previously noted, *in vitro,* that isolated bloodless perfused canine kidneys can release significant levels of renin in the absence of a functioning adrenal gland[14]. This finding, along with our present observations in anephric hypertensive man (Table 6), suggests further independence, for some causes of hypertension, from the renin–aldosterone–angiotensin system.

SUMMARY AND CONCLUSIONS

Plasma renin and erythropoietin (ESF) levels have been measured in 45 uremic patients. These patients were studied prior to institution of dietary control, fluid and sodium restriction, and intermittent hemodialysis. Follow-up observations were possible in most instances after therapy and after bilateral nephrectomy. Some patients were normotensive, but others were hypertensive (diastolic blood pressure greater than 100 mm Hg).

Significant levels of plasma renin and ESF were found in uremic man. Sustained hypertension after dialysis in patients with renal insufficiency is usually associated with elevated renin levels. Although it has been reported that in some instances bilateral nephrectomy results in lowering of renin levels as well as blood pressure, our findings indicate that hypertension can persist in anephric man without elevated renin levels. Moreover, elevated renin or renin-like substances were noted in anephric patients who were normotensive.

These findings indicate that some causes of hypertension, particularly in anephric man, do not operate through the renin–aldosterone–angiotension sstemy. Also, the present study confirms previous observations that extrarenal renin or renin-like substances do exist to a significant degree in man. Furthermore, ESF is also present in uremic and anephric man, but the levels are not relatable to the presence or absence of hypertension. In addition, factors controlling the regulation of extrarenal renin and extrarenal ESF in anephric man do not appear to be similar.

ACKNOWLEDGMENTS

These studies were in large part fostered and supported by Dr. W. W. Scott. The initial observation on extrarenal ESF in man was made in 1967 at the Johns Hopkins–Stellenbosch Transplant Center in South Africa fostered by Dr. Scott.

We appreciate the helpful assistance of Phyllis Williams, Virginia Juliano, Janet Kellham, Joyce Jividen, Andre Bulba, and Edmund Dynwinski during this study.

REFERENCES

1. Gordon, A. S. Hemopoietin. *Physiol. Rev.* **39**:1–40, 1959.
2. Wilkinson, R., Scott, D. F., Uldall, P. R., Kerr, D. N. S., and Swinney, J. Plasma renin and exchangeable sodium in the hypertension of chronic renal failure. *Quart. J. Med.* **39**:377–394, 1970.
3. Murphy, G. P., Mirand, E. A., and Kenny, G. M. Erythropoietin alterations in uremia renoprival states and after renal allograft. *Urol. Digest* **9**:24–32, 1970.
4. Mirand, E. A., and Murphy, G. P. Erythropoietin alterations in patients with uremia renal allografts, or without kidneys. *J.A.M.A.* **209**:392–398, 1969.
5. Gunnells, J. C., Grim, C. E., Robinson, R. R., and Wilderman, B. S. Plasma renin activity in healthy subjects and patients with hypertension. *Arch. Int. Med.* **119**:232, 1967.
6. Weintraub, A. H., Gordon, A. S., Becker, E. L., Camiscoli, J. F., and Contrera, J. F. *Am. J. Physiol.* **207**:523, 1964.

7. Fisher, J. W., Hatch, F. E., Roh, B. L., Allen, R. C., and Kelly, B. J. Erythropoietin inhibitor in kidney extracts and plasma from anemic uremic human subjects. *Blood* **31**:440, 1968.
8. Mirand, E. A., Murphy, G. P., Steeves, R. A., Groenewald, J. H., and DeKlerk, J. N. Erythropoietin activity in anephric allotransplanted unilaterally nephrectomized and intact man. *J. Lab. Clin. Med.* **73**:121–128, 1969.
9. Hampres, C. L., Skillman, J. J., Lyons, J. M., Olsen, J. E., and Merrill, J. P. *Circulation* **35**:272, 1967.
10. Hegstrom, R. M., Murray, J. S., Pendras, J. P., Burnell, J. M., and Scribner, B. M. *Trans. Am. Soc. Artif. Int. Organs* **8**:266, 1962.
11. Onesti, G., Swartz, G., Ramirez, O., and Breast, A. N. *Trans Am. Soc. Artif. Int. Organs* **14**:361, 1968.
12. Vertes, V., Cangiano, M. D., Berman, L. B., and Gould, A. *New Engl. J. Med.* **281**:272, 1969.
13. Toussaint, C. *New Engl. J. Med.* **281**:272, 1969.
14. Smolev, J. K., Baer, D. M., and Murphy, G. P. Renin release and utilization by the isolated canine kidney. *J. Urol.* **106**:163, 1971.

Measurement of Renal Vein Renins or Differential Renal Function Studies in the Diagnosis of Curable, Renovascular Hypertension?*

Thomas A. Stamey†

Measurements of plasma renin activity are now widely used in the evaluation of patients with potentially curable renovascular hypertension, and justifiably so. But a short decade ago, differential renal function studies were received with equal enthusiasm. What are the relative merits of these two methodologies? Because my first research efforts under the guidance of Dr. William Wallace Scott were in the field of renovascular hypertension, I have chosen this subject as my part of the Festschrift in his honor.

We have used both differential renal function studies and measurements of plasma renin activity in the evaluation of our hypertensive patients during the past few years. Using the renin method of Boucher[1], and the technique of differential function studies described earlier[2,3], we can make the following general comparisons:

The advantages of measurement of renal vein renins over differential function studies are that (a) samples can be collected with relative ease and safety and (b) renin determinations are the only way to asscess the significance of unilaterally small kidneys with parenchymal disease but normal main renal arteries.

*Supported by U.S. Public Health Service Training Grant No. 5 TOI AM 05513.
†Professor of Surgery, Chairman Division of Urology, Stanford University School of Medicine, Stanford, California.

The disadvantages of using renin activities are (a) the complexity and coefficient of variation of the renin assay, (b) the substantial influence of diet, antihypertensive medications, and position of the patient on the level of renin activity, and (c) the undeniable fact that differential renal vein renins yield no information regarding vascular disease or renal function in the contralateral kidney.

I shall now consider these points in greater detail and present some informative data from three patients.

COLLECTION OF SAMPLES

Perhaps the major reason measurement of renal vein renins will ultimately prevail over differential renal function studies is the ease and safety of collecting renal vein blood. With a fluoroscope and Seldinger catheter, one can catheterize the femoral vein, pass a curved catheter into one renal vein, and later move to the contralateral vein. Provided the patients are observed for a few hours following catheter withdrawal, the procedure can be performed on an outpatient basis. By contrast, differential renal function studies cannot be done on outpatients. More importantly, function studies have never been popular because they are lengthy and demand careful attention to technical detail for an adequate study. Including the saddle anesthesia, equilibration time, and collection of samples which show reproducible differences in consecutive periods, about 3 hr is required for a good function study. Since two prostatectomies can be done in the same period of time, it is understandable that function studies have never been financially rewarding. Furthermore, although the morbidity resulting from differential function studies has been insignificant (especially if the large ureteral catheters are left indwelling until the following day), renal vein catheterization is clearly more comfortable and acceptable to the patient than ureteral catheterization.

As appealing as this argument seems for using renal vein renins, the potential errors in the collection of renal vein blood must be remembered. In the best studies, these errors are monitored. Contrast agents, because of their potential influence on renin secretion, should not be injected into the renal veins to check placement of the venous catheter prior to sample withdrawal; in fact, since one catheter is always used to draw blood from both left and right renal veins, contrast should not be injected after collection from the first vein lest the sodium and osmotic influence of the contrast agent reduce renin activity in the contralateral kidney. Only after both left and right renal vein samples have been drawn should both veins be injected to visualize the placement of the catheter. This is clearly a disadvantage in the case of the first vein because a second catheterization may not end up in the identical position of the first withdrawal. An experienced radiologist can usually tell whether the catheter is in the renal vein by fluoroscopy.

THE VALUE OF THE PAH EXTRACTION RATIO

Even when the catheter is within the renal vein, one may withdraw some nonrenal venous blood; therefore, we always compare the extraction of *p*-aminohippurate (PAH) in the left and right renal venous samples. This is easily done by giving the patient half of a 10-ml ampule of 20% PAH by intravenous injection and by placing the remaining 5 ml in a continuous intravenous infusion of 5% dextrose in water. The rate of infusion, provided it is reasonably constant, is not important. We then determine the concentration of PAH in all three samples that are submitted for assay of renin activity: the left and right renal vein plasma, and the plasma from the inferior vena cava. We reported in 1963 that in humans with unilateral Goldblatt kidneys[3], as Phillips *et al*[4]. had previously shown in dogs, ischemia does not reduce the capability of the renal tubular cells to completely extract PAH from peritubular blood into the urine. Thus, any difference in the extraction ratio of PAH in the left and right renal veins is indicative of nonrenal venous blood in the sample with the lower extraction ratio. About one third of our renal vein samples have shown a significant difference (greater than 10%) in the extraction of PAH, which has led us to be cautious in interpreting differences in renin activity in these patients. The major sources of nonrenal venous blood from catheters that lie well within the renal veins are (a) the ovarian or testicular vein on the left and (b) the suction of vena caval blood into the right renal venous catheter in the presence of reduced venous blood flow. I would urge the adoption of the PAH extraction ratio as the ideal physiological way to check the accuracy of renal venous sampling. Indeed, even injection of contrast under positive pressure through the catheter at the completion of the last renal vein sample is clearly not representative of those physical forces present at the time negative pressure is applied to withdraw the blood sample.

ACCURACY OF RENIN ACTIVITY MEASUREMENTS COMPARED WITH PAH CONCENTRATION INDICES OF EXCESSIVE WATER REABSORPTION

The identification of unilateral renal ischemia by differential renal function studies depends upon urine flow rate differences that are accompanied by a substantial increase in the reabsorption of water. For patients with segmental disease, the increase in PAH concentration has varied between 26 and 92% (Table 1), depending upon the size of the ischemic segment; for main renal artery obstruction, in the absence of renal infarction,

**Table 1. Functional Characteristics of Segmental Renal Ischemia in the
Presence of Urea, Saline, and Antidiuretic Hormone[a]**

Case No.	Urine flow (ml/min)			U_{PAH} (mg %)			C_{PAH}[b] (ml/min)			U_{sodium}		
	I	C	I/C	I	C	I/C	I	C	I/C	I	C	I/C
1	0.5	1.8	0.28	424	290	1.46	99	240	0.41	37	79	0.47
2	4.7	7.5	0.63	103	68	1.51	249	262	0.95	71	82	0.87
3	4.7	7.0	0.67[c]	152	117	1.32	226	276	0.82	94	90	1.07
4	3.8	7.6	0.50[d]	87	57	1.53	226	301	0.75	48	65	0.74
5	4.5	8.5	0.52	75	54	1.38	165	227	0.73	53	52	1.01
6	2.8	5.8	0.48	245	199	1.28	135	219	0.61	73	80	0.92
7	4.7	12.8	0.37	96	50	1.92	196	278	0.71	100	104	0.96
8	1.0	3.6	0.28	236	157	1.51	125	303	0.41	131	184	0.94
9	2.9	5.5	0.53	140	121	1.40	168	272	0.62	96	100	0.96
10[e]	3.8	7.0	0.54	113	67	1.67	212	234	0.91	38	60	0.63
11	2.7	8.6	0.32	87	66	1.31	182	446	0.41	46	35	1.32
12	1.4	4.5	0.30	125	99	1.26	97	252	0.38	103	109	0.94
Average			0.45			1.46			0.64			0.90

[a] I, ischemic kidney; C, contralateral kidney.
[b] Corrected to 1.73 m².
[c] Study done under oral water diuresis.
[d] Study done under general anesthesia.
[e] A nephrectomy was performed in all patients except No. 10, who had a simple cyst unroofed.

the increase in PAH concentration has varied between 100 and > 1000%. The standard deviation of determining PAH concentration is small, 5% or less, and even less when replicate samples of urine are determined in an autoanalyzer.

By contrast, one standard deviation of the Boucher method is about 10–20% of the mean, depending somewhat on the level of renin activity in the sample[5].

The error depends on a number of complicated factors, such as correction of the plasma for the hematocrit, the 3-hr incubation, the absorption and later extraction from a cation exchange resin, and the final technique of assay in the rat. To be sure, the error can be reduced by using a rigidly controlled four-point bioassay and, in the case of renal vein and inferior vena caval samples, by assaying all three serially in the same rat at a time when the rat is stable. Despite these precautions, renin activity measurements are no contest when compared to the simple chemical determination of PAH. The latter is available in the simplest hospital laboratory[3], whereas renin measurements remain largely confined to sophisticated research laboratories. Hopefully, immunoassay techniques[6] will improve both the accuracy and the availability of renin determinations.

FACTORS INFLUENCING RENIN ACTIVITY IN PERIPHERAL AND RENAL VENOUS BLOOD

The concentration of renin in peripheral plasma, and therefore presumably in the renal vein, is influenced substantially (severalfold) by posture[7], the time of day or night[8], sodium balance[9], surgery[10], and various antihypertensive drugs including diuretics[11], hydralazine[12], and methyldopa[13]. Indeed, Hunt and his colleagues feel that only guanethidine fails to alter differential renal vein renin in the diagnosis of a renin-secreting kidney responsible for hypertension[14].

These factors that so markedly change renin concentration, as well as the substantial errors in the bioassay method, would not be so important if a severalfold difference in renal vein concentrations was diagnostic of curable, unilateral renal disease. Most authors, however, report that a 1.5 ratio difference (renin activity of operated kidney/renin activity of non-operated kidney) correlates with cure of the hypertension[15,16]. The very careful study of Gunnells et al.[17], however, is interesting. Of 25 operated-on patients, the 16 who were cured or improved had a mean ratio of 4.49 ± 1.53 and an elevated peripheral plasma renin; the nine surgical failures had a mean ratio of 2.34 ± 0.54 and their peripheral plasma renins were normal. Surely, if the error of determination has a 10–20% coefficient of variation in 66% of replicate samples (and a 20–40% variation [2 SD] in the remaining 34%), ratio errors in opposite direction can easily approach the diagnostic ratio of 1.5.

THE ADVANTAGE OF SODIUM DEPLETION BEFORE COLLECTION OF RENAL VENOUS SAMPLES

More important, however, than the potential assay errors in measuring renal vein renin differences is the demonstration by Hunt's group at the Mayo Clinic[14] that sodium depletion increases the diagnostic sensitivity of the ratio differences in venous renin activity. Specifically, studies in 41 sodium-depleted patients were predictive of surgical cure in 90% but were predictive in only 35% of 26 patients who were on a normal sodium diet. Other investigators use upright posture to stimulate renin from the Goldblatt kidney[18] and thereby increase the diagnostic difference between the two renal veins.

Why does renin stimulation, whether by low sodium diet[14], posture[18], hydralazine infusion[12], or acute blood pressure decrease by infusion of nitroprusside[19], increase the renin activity in the Goldblatt kidney more than it influences the renin activity in the contralateral kidney? It has been known for years from work in animals that tissue renin disappears from the contralateral, nonischemic kidney as it accumulates in the experimental

Goldblatt kidney[20]. For this reason, in the human with unilateral renovascular hypertension, the renin activity in the vein from the contralateral
kidney is the same as the activity in the blood entering the renal artery,
suggesting no addition of renin during passage through the kidney. Occasionally, the activity is *less* in the contralateral renal vein than in the
inferior vena caval sample (representative of aortic blood activity), perhaps
indicating extraction into renal lymph or urine; these latter differences,
however, are usually so small that they are well within the error of the assay
methodology. It is clear, nevertheless, that in the unilateral Goldblatt
situation the only renin circulating is from the Goldblatt kidney. For this
reason, stimulation of renin secretion by any method accentuates differences
in renal vein renin values. In our unit, renal vein renin samples are never
collected unless the patient has been on a 10-mEq sodium diet for at least
7 days. We measure the 24-hr urine sodium at the time the renal vein samples
are collected so that the degree of sodium depletion is known.

THE DISADVANTAGE OF SODIUM DEPLETION BEFORE
DIFFERENTIAL RENAL FUNCTION STUDIES

While the evidence is clear that a low sodium diet stimulates renin and
increases the diagnostic usefulness of renal vein renins[14], a low sodium
level in the urine prevents excessive water reabsorption and thereby blunts
the diagnostic increase in PAH or inulin concentration from the Goldblatt
kidney. Thus, the patient must be salt-repleted after renal vein renin col-
lections before differential function studies are performed.

For example, R. R., a 49-year-old white man, presented at Stanford in
late 1969 with malignant hypertension (hemorrhages and exudate in the
fundi with early papilledema and 4 + proteinuria). The serum sodium upon
admission was 129 mEq/liter and the serum creatinine 1.7 mg/100 ml. He
was placed on a 2.0-g sodium diet. Intravenous Aldomet (methyldopa)
during the first 24 hr, followed by 500 mg by mouth every 6 hr, produced
a good blood pressure response. Angiography revealed a severe right renal
artery stenosis and a normal left renal artery (Fig. 1). On November 10,
1969, differential renal function studies were performed, about 1 week after
admission (Table 2). His serum sodium at the time was 134 mEq/liter.
He was discharged on Aldomet 500 mg four times a day without salt restriction. He returned 5 weeks later, showed an 8-lb weight gain, and had a serum
sodium of 139 mEq/liter with a serum creatinine of 1.5 mg/100 ml. Differential renal function studies were repeated on December 22, 1969 (Table 2),
when his serum sodium was 140 mEq/liter. Aldomet therapy was not withheld
during either function study. He received an intravenous infusion of 8%
urea in saline at 10 ml/min during both function studies; the serum urea

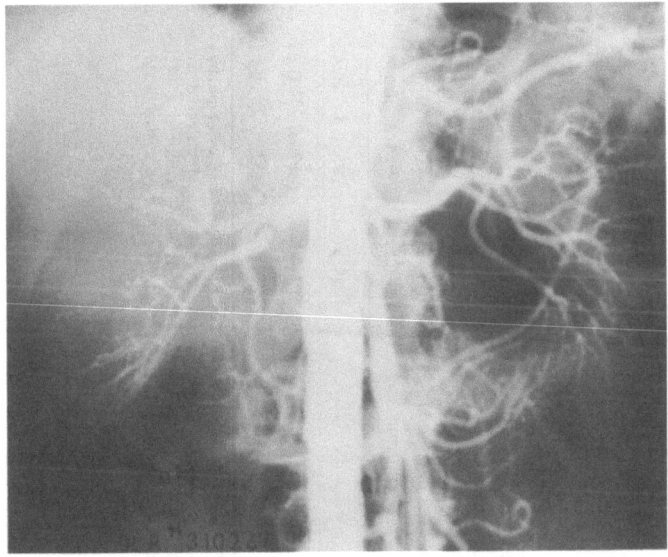

Fig. 1. Angiogram in R. R., a 49-year-old white man with malignant hypertension. The right renal artery shows severe narrowing from atherosclerotic disease at the renal artery ostium. The left renal artery is normal.

nitrogen, from the infusion, was 85 mg/100 ml at the beginning of the first collection period in the first study (November 10, 1969) and 83 mg/100 ml in the second study (December 22, 1969). Despite the osmotic load of urea, urinary sodium was only 5–7 mEq/liter during the first function study (Table 2). During this study, and despite a marked difference in GFR and RPF, there was no excessive water reabsorption as measured by inulin and creatinine concentration (ratio, R/L = 0.96). In the second study, however, with a serum sodium of 140 mEq/liter and an *identical* difference in GFR and RPF, excessive water reabsorption was substantial (ratio inulin concentration, R/L = 3.04). Since the GFR was unchanged in the second study, the excessive water reabsorption produced a 17:1 difference in urine flow rate compared with a 6:1 ratio in the first study. In the first study, the 6:1 difference in urine flow rate simply reflected the disparity in GFR. Because the only difference in these two studies was severe sodium depletion during the first study, and because the osmotic load from urea was identical in both studies, it is reasonable to believe that in the absence of adequate sodium in the nephron, excessive water reabsorption is limited or even absent. Lastly, the greater sensitivity of differences in PAH concentration than that of inulin or creatinine is readily apparent in Table 2. Both this finding and the

Table 2. R. R., 49-Year-Old White Man with Right Renal Artery Stenosis (Fig. 1)

Date	Urine flow (ml/min)			Inulin concentration (mg/100 ml)			Inulin clearance (ml/min)			PAH concentration (mg/100 ml)			PAH clearance (ml/min)			Urine sodium (mEq/liter)			Filtration fraction		
	R	L	R/L	R	L	R/L	R	L	R/L	R	L	R/L	R	L	R/L	R	L	R/L	R	L	R/L
11/10/69	0.7	4.3	0.17	173	181	0.96	6	41	0.15	180	116	1.55	38	151	0.25	7	5	1.40	0.17	0.27	0.63
12/22/69	0.5	8.7	0.06	236	78	3.04	7	42	0.17	264	52	5.08	41	148	0.28	23	29	0.79	0.17	0.28	0.61

[a] Differential renal function studies, using an infusion of 8% urea in saline, were performed during salt restriction (11/10/69) and after partial salt repletion (12/22/69). While GFR and RPF were virtually the same in both studies, differences in urine flow rate (6:1) reflected the disparity in GFR during salt restriction. With adequate sodium in the nephrons on 12/22/69, excessive water reabsorption produced a 17:1 difference in urine flow rate. The greater sensitivity of PAH over inulin or creatinine concentrations as a measure of excessive water reabsorption and the characteristic difference in filtration fractions have been described previously[21].

characteristic difference in filtration fraction have been previously discussed[21].

Peripheral vein renin values were determined twice before surgery and immediately prior to the induction of anesthesia for a saphenous vein bypass graft. These data, along with the tissue renin values at the time of surgery and the dramatic postoperative fall in peripheral vein renin activity, are presented in Table 3.

THE QUANTITATIVE VALUE OF URETERAL CATHETERIZATION STUDIES FOR MEASURING EXCESSIVE WATER REABSORPTION, FOR OBSERVING THE RENAL FUNCTION OF EACH KIDNEY, AND FOR ESTIMATING THE PRESENCE OF NONFILTERING ISCHEMIC SEGMENTS

A good way to observe the relative merits of renal vein renin values and differential renal function studies is to compare them in the same patient. I have chosen a 36-year-old white man with a segmental lesion because ischemic segments that involve only a part of one kidney are the most difficult to detect. G. S. was first seen at Stanford in April 1969, 4 weeks after the discovery of high blood pressure (220 mm Hg systolic) during an examination for acute appendicitis. His blood pressure was normal in 1967. Upon admission his blood pressure was 170/130 mm Hg, his serum creatinine was 1.1 mg/100 ml, and his electrolytes were normal. Neither the fundi nor the urinalysis were remarkable. The intravenous urogram showed equal

Table 3. Renin Activity in the Peripheral Vein, Renal Vein, and Renal Tissue
of R. R., a 49-Year-Old White Man with Right Renal Artery
Stenosis and Malignant Hypertension

Time	Source	Renin activity[a] $(m\mu g/100 \ ml)$
12/24/69	Peripheral[b]	1,950
12/28/69	Peripheral	2,560
12/29/69	Surgery	
	Preanesthesia	1,820
	L renal vein	3,190
	R renal vein	20,220
	Aorta	4,030
	L renal tissue	1,400. $(m\mu g/g)$
	R renal tissue	81,500. $(m\mu g/g)$
12/30/69	Peripheral	200
12/31/69	Peripheral	160
1/8/70	Peripheral	490

[a] Boucher method[1].
[b] Peripheral vein renin activity in normotensive controls in our laboratory, depending on position and time of day, varies between 200 and 600 mμg/100 ml.

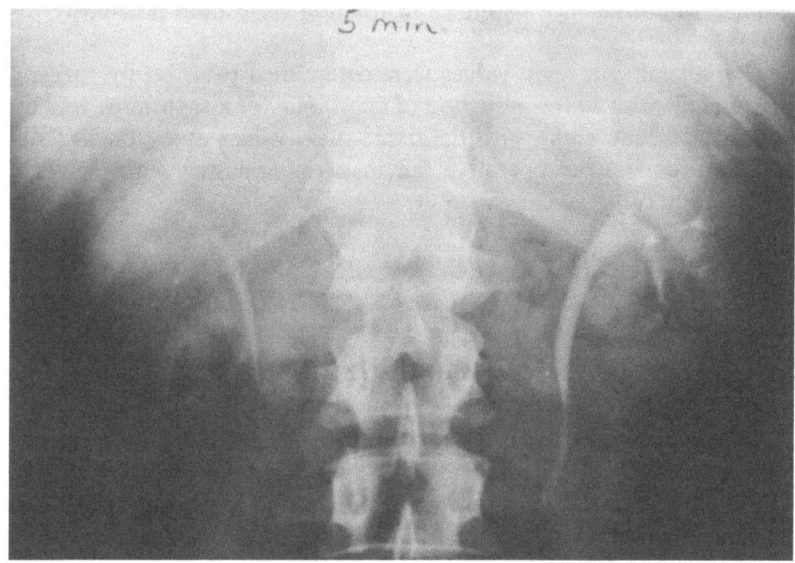

Fig. 2. A 5-min intravenous urogram in G. S., a 36-year-old white man with hypertension. Earlier 1-, 2-, and 3-min sequence films showed equal appearance time, but the volume of contrast excretion is clearly less in the right kidney.

appearance time in early films, but less volume of contrast in the right kidney than in the left (Fig. 2). The hippuran-I^{131} renogram showed a delayed excretory phase in the right kidney (Fig. 3). Angiograms (Fig. 4 and 5) indicated three renal arteries to the right kidney with a peculiar dilatation in the middle, largest artery. On a 10-mEq sodium diet, peripheral vein and renal vein renin samples were drawn in the supine position and, after 15 mins, in the upright position (Table 4). The ratio difference was 1.6, with no increase in the upright position. Because the patient had a severe allergic reaction following the angiography, contrast was not injected into the renal veins after the collection of the samples. The extraction ratios for

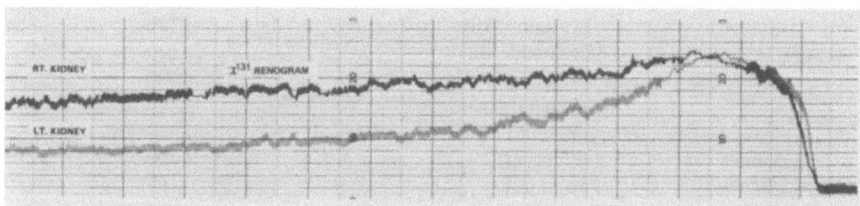

Fig. 3. A hippuran-I^{131} renogram in G. S. The delayed excretory phase, in the absence of obstruction and in the presence of pelvic symmetry (Fig. 2), is diagnostic of a disproportionate reduction in urinary excretion in relation to renal mass.

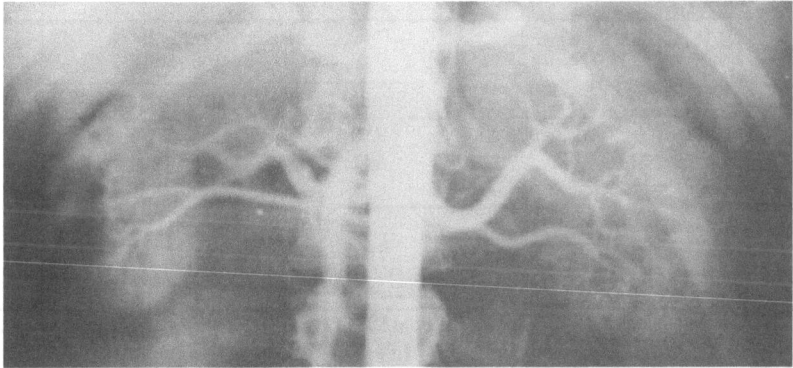

Fig. 4. Early phase angiogram in G. S. There are three arteries to the right kidney; the middle and largest appears dilated and irregular. The left renal artery is normal.

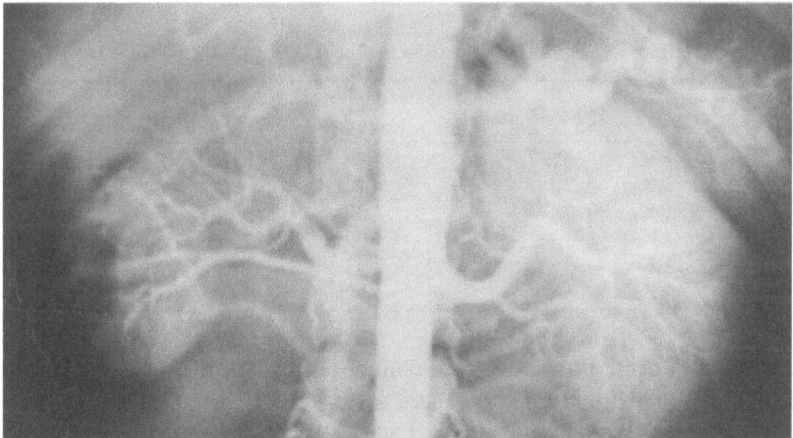

Fig. 5. A later phase angiogram in G. S. The nephrogram is best in the lower pole of the right kidney. Note that the right kidney is only slightly smaller than the left. At nephrectomy, it weighed 110 g. Thus, a gross disparity existed between renal mass and urine flow rate differences (Table 6), which suggested large areas of renal tissue that contributed no glomerular filtrate.

PAH, however, were the same in both kidneys (Table 5), indicating the absence of nonrenal venous blood. Following salt repletion, differential renal function studies were performed during saddle anesthesia and the intravenous infusion of urea and saline. Three consecutive 10-min periods were collected after equilibration of inulin and PAH. The differences in urine flow rate showed perfect agreement (Table 6), indicating a substantial

Table 4. Segmental Renal Ischemia (G. S., 36-Year-Old Male)

	Renal vein Penin (mμg/100 ml)			
	Supine	R/L	Upright	R/L
R kidney	951		2076	
L Kidney	608	1.6	1404	1.5
Peripheral			1420	

Table 5. Segmental Renal Ischemia (G.S., 36-Year-Old Male)

	renal vein PAH (mg/100 ml)		PAH extraction ratio (%)	
	Supine	Upright	Supine	Upright
R kidney	0.17	0.17	89	90
L kidney	0.15	0.15	91	91
Peripheral	1.60	1.70		

Table 6. Segmental Renal Ischemia (G. S., 36-Year-Old Male)

	Urine flow (ml/min)	R/L
RK$_1$	1.46	
LK$_1$	4.78	0.31
RK$_2$	1.30	
LK$_2$	4.00	0.33
RK$_3$	1.32	
LK$_3$	4.62	0.29

disparity in urine flow rate when compared to the differences in renal mass (Fig. 5). Renal function differences are averaged for the three consecutive periods and presented in Table 7. Excessive water reabsorption was present, as indicated by the 1.26 ratio of PAH concentration (Table 7), which is at the lower limits of the diagnostic range for segmental renal ischemia (Table 1). Thus, both the renal vein renin ratios and the PAH concentration diff-

Table 7. Segmental Renal Ischemia (G. S., 36-Year-Old Male)

Urine flow (ml/min)	U$_{PAH}$ (mg %)	U$_{IN}$ (mg %)	U$_{Na}$ (mEq/L)	C$_{PAH}$ (ml/min /1.73 m^2)	C$_{IN}$ (ml/min /1.73 m^2)
RK 1.4	RK 125	RK 235	RK 103	RK 97	RK 24
LK 4.5	LK 99	LK 191	LK 109	LK 252	LK 63
R/L 0.30	R/L 1.26	R/L 1.23	R/L 0.94	R/L 0.38	R/L 0.82

erences were suggestive of renal ischemia, but only the PAH indicated excessive water reabsorption in the range of segmental disease. Moreover, we learned from the function studies that renal plasma flow was 252 ml/min in the contralateral kidney and surprisingly low (97 ml/min) in the right kidney with multiple main renal arteries. Sodium differences, as usual in segmental disease, were minimal. Most important, however, was the disparity in urine flow rate differences (3:1) and estimations of renal mass differences (less than 2:1), which suggested large areas of renal tissue that did not contribute to urine flow. A nephrectomy was performed on April 21, 1969; the kidney weighed 110 g. Large areas in the middle half of the kidney showed crowded glomeruli and atrophic tubules. Only the middle one of the three arteries showed disease: fibromuscular dysplasia with subintimal dissection. His blood pressure was 140/90–95 mm Hg 4 weeks after surgery. A report from his physician in October 1970 indicated his blood pressure was 140/100 during an insurance physical, with repeat readings of 135/90 and 120/80 mm Hg. We examined him on 25 March 1971; his blood pressure was 140/105 mm Hg both lying and standing. His fundi and urine were normal.

In this patient, all investigations were positive: in the intravenous pyelogram, although the appearance time was equal, the 5-min film suggested less contrast excretion in the right kidney (Fig. 2); the renogram was positive (Fig. 3), especially so in view of the bilateral pelvic symmetry (Fig. 2); the arteriogram showed multiple arteries to the right kidney with disease in one (Fig. 5); renin ratio differences (1.6) localized to the right kidney (Table 4) but in the range of main renal arterial disease; the function studies (Table 7) were reproducible, positive for segmental ischemia, and indicated a borderline blood flow to the contralateral kidney. Which study showed the greatest disparity?

The most impressive finding to me, especially in view of the potential methodological errors just reviewed, was the 3:1 difference in urine flow rates (Table 6) from kidneys that clearly had less than a 2:1 difference in renal mass; indeed, the right kidney weighed 110 g. Without bladder leakage and with reproducible differences in urine flow rate, there had to be significant renal mass that was not contributing to glomerular filtrate. The additional finding of excessive water reabsorption within our reported range of segmental lesions[22], and the knowledge that the contralateral renal plasma flow was borderline, surely represented more quantitative data than obtained by the intravenous urogram, the renogram, and renal vein renin values. Moreover, who would have guessed the extent of the disparity in GFR and urine flow rate in the right kidney? Certainly no one would have guessed the disparity from the intravenous urogram, the arteriogram, or the renal vein renin values.

THE UNIQUE ROLE OF RENAL VEIN RENINS IN THE
ASSESSMENT OF UNILATERAL PARENCHYMAL DISEASE IN
THE PRESENCE OF NORMAL MAIN RENAL ARTERIES

In the past 5 years, every patient with positive differential renal function studies characteristic of main renal artery lesions has also had a positive ratio (> 2.0) in renal vein renin activities *provided* renin was stimulated by either low sodium diet or surgery.

On the other hand, unilateral parenchymal disease—especially pyelonephritis—in the presence of normal main renal arteries is very difficult to evaluate. Not only may severe ischemic segments produce insufficient glomerular filtrate for the detection of excessive water reabsorption, but even in the presence of filtration, excessive water reabsorption in the cortical areas of the nephron may be diluted by the medullary failure to reabsorb water. As clearly illustrated by Fair[23], nonfiltering ischemic segments in the absence of pyelonephritis can be detected by comparing the ratio of renal mass to the ratio of GFR, RPF, or even urine flow (as, for example, in G. S.). However, all nephrons in a pyelonephritic kidney must pass through the diseased medulla, an area characterized by failure to reabsorb sodium and water[24].

We have one patient with documented unilateral pyelonephritis and a "water-losing" pattern on differential function studies who is still normotensive 5 years after nephrectomy. Because renal vein renins were diagnostic of ischemia before surgery, and because renal biopsies at the time of surgery confirmed the absence of tissue renin in the contralateral kidney, her studies are presented in detail. D. S. was 30 years old when first seen in 1966. She had a 12-year history of recurrent chills, fever, and right flank pain accompanied by positive urine cultures. Hypertension (170/120) was first discovered in 1960 during her third and last pregnancy. Despite various antihypertensive medications, the blood pressure remained about the same. Urinary symptoms were controlled by constant sulfonamide therapy. When we first examined her, her urine sediment was normal, and a urine culture was sterile 14 days after stopping sulfonamide therapy. The serum creatinine was 1.1 mg/100 ml. An intravenous urogram was consistent with right pyelonephritis (Fig. 6), and an angiogram showed bilaterally normal renal arteries (Fig. 7). Renal vein and inferior vena caval samples were collected on October 25, 1966, while she was on a normal sodium diet (Table 8); differential function studies were performed on October 26, 1966, with an infusion of 8% urea in saline (Table 9); and a right nephroureterectomy with left renal biopsy was carried out on November 2, 1966. Renal tissue renin values were determined on the surgical specimens (Table 8). This patient has been seen repeatedly over the past 5 years because of several bladder

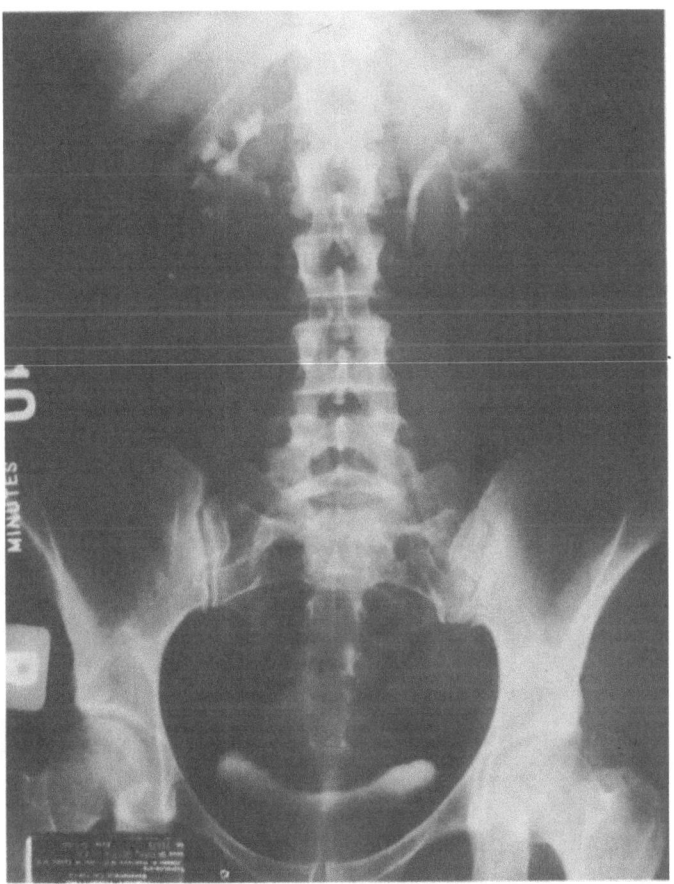

Fig. 6. A 10-min intravenous urogram in D. S., a 30-year-old white woman with a 10-year history of chills, fever, and right flank pain secondary to documented urinary infections. The calyceal distortion and size of the right kidney are suggestive of pyelonephritic damage.

infections due to varying organisms, but her blood pressure has always been 120–130/80 mm Hg.

The renal function data (Table 9) show a characteristic water- and sodium-losing lesion in the right kidney, similar in every way to studies performed on normotensive patients with unilateral renal infection. Observe, however, that the 3:1 or 4:1 difference in urine flow rate and renal function (GFR and RPF) is approximately proportional to the estimated difference in renal mass (Fig. 7). Not surprisingly, the right kidney weighed 64 g at nephrectomy. Thus, nonfiltering ischemic segments do not enter into this

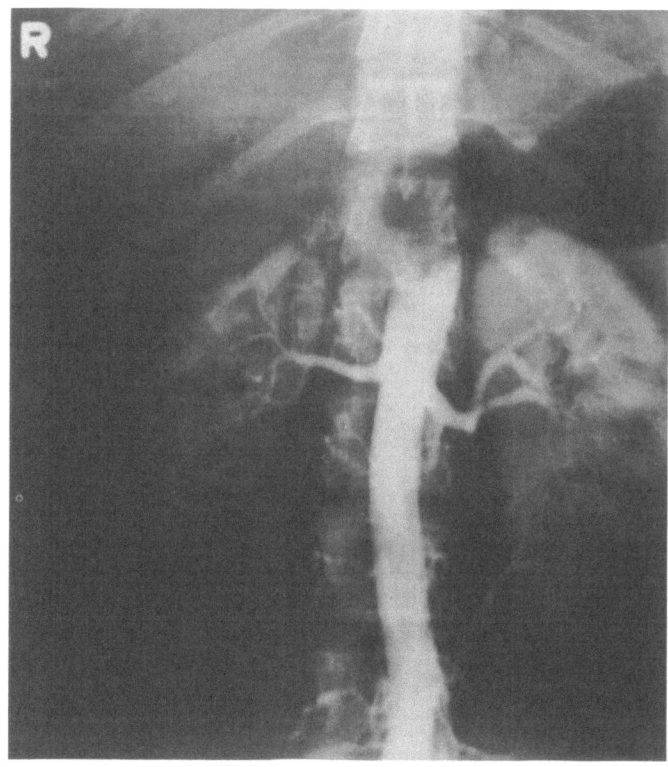

Fig. 7. An angiogram in D. S., showing irregularity in the cortical border of
the right kidney. The left kidney measured 15.0 cm and the right 10.5 cm.
At nephrectomy, the right kidney weighed 64 g. Unlike G. S. (Fig. 2–5), the
disparity in renal mass in D. S. approximates the differences in renal function and urine excretion (Table 9).

**Table 8. Renin Activity in the Renal Veins, Inferior Vena Cava, and Renal
Tissue of D. S., a 30-Year-Old White Woman with
Unilateral, Right Pyelonephritis**

Time	Source	Rein activity[a] (mμg/100 ml)	
10/25/66	R renal vein	4,270	
	L renal vein	2,640	
	Inferior vena cava	2,470	
11/2/66	R renal cortex	12,230	(mμg/g)
	L renal cortex	0	(mμg/g)

[a] Boucher method[1].

Table 9. Three Consecutive Collection Periods in D. S., a 30-Year-Old White Woman with Hypertension and Unilateral, Right Pyelonephritis

	Urine flow[a] (ml/min)			Inulin concentration (mg/100 ml)			Inulin clearance (ml/min)			PAH Concentration (mg/100 ml)			PAH clearance (ml/min)			Urine sodium (mEq/liter)			Filtration fraction		
	R	L	R/L	R	L	R/L	R	L	R/L	R	L	R/L	R	L	R/L	R	L	R/L	R	L	R/L
1st period	3.7	12.3	0.30	80	102	0.78	18	76	0.24	31	42	0.74	120	543	0.22	78	73	1.07	0.15	0.14	1.07
2nd period	4.4	17.4	0.25	67	89	0.75	18	94	0.19	27	37	0.73	125	676	0.19	80	75	1.07	0.14	0.14	1.00
3rd period	4.9	16.1	0.30	61	86	0.71	18	84	0.21	24	35	0.69	128	592	0.22	79	74	1.07	0.14	0.14	1.00
Average	4.3	15.3	0.28	69	92	0.75	18	85	0.21	27	38	0.71	124	604	0.21	79	74	1.07	0.14	0.14	1.00

[a] These studies were performed with an intravenous infusion of 8% urea in saline.

diagnosis as they do in patient G. S. (Table 4–7 and Figures 2–5). Moreover, microscopic examination of the right kidney in D. S. showed thyroid-like tubules, tubular casts, and inflammation around the pelvis but no evidence of crowded glomeruli, tubular atrophy, or prominent juxtaglomerular cells.

D. S., then, seems clearly documented as a patient with unilateral pyelonephritis with neither excretory functional nor histological evidence of renal ischemia. The right renal vein renin activity, however, was 1.6 times that of the left, and, at surgery, the absence of tissue renin in the contra-lateral left kidney (Table 8) was further confirmation of a renin-producing right kidney. Thus, the determination of renal vein renin activity may be of critical importance in assessing unilateral parenchymal disease in the presence of normal renal arteries.

In conclusion, it seems to me that if a medical center has the organization and interested urologists who can perform careful, reproducible differential renal function studies, the information obtained from these studies in 95% of hypertensive patients is more valuable than that obtained by measurement of renal vein renin activity. Patients like D. S. with unilateral parenchymal disease and normal renal arteries are an important exception.

On the other hand, where this interest and organization are absent—which unfortunately includes the great majority of centers—the determination of renal vein renins during low sodium stimulation offers the physician an important opportunity to determine which kidney is the most ischemic.

REFERENCES

1. Boucher, R., Veyrat, R., de Champlain, J., and Genest, J. New procedures for measurement of human plasma angiotensin and renin activity levels. *Canad. Med. Assoc. J.* **90**: 194, 1964.
2. Stamey, T. A., Nudelman, I. J., Good. P. H., Schwentker, F. N., and Hendricks, F. Functional characteristics of renovascular hypertension. *Medicine* **40**:347, 1961.
3. Stamey, T. A. *Renovascular Hypertension,* Williams and Wilkins, Baltimore, 1963.
4. Phillips, R. A., Dole, V. P., Hamilton, P. B., Emerson, K., Jr., Archibald, R. M., and Van Slyke, D. D. Effects of acute hemorrhagic and traumatic shock on renal function of dogs. *Am. J. Physiol.* **145**:314, 1946.
5. Assaykeen, T. A., Otsuka, K., and Ganong, W. F. Rate of disappearance of exogenous dog renin from the plasma of nephrectomized dogs. *Proc. Soc. Exptl. Biol. Med.* **127**: 306, 1968.
6. Boyd, G. W., Fitz, A. E., Adamson, A. R., and Peart, W. S. Radioimmunoassay determination of plasma-renin activity. *Lancet* **2**:213, 1969.
7. Cohen, E. L., Conn, J. W., and Rovner, D. R. Postural augmentation of plasma renin activity and aldosterone excretion in normal people. *J. Clin. Invest.* **46**:418, 1967.
8. Gordon, R. D., Wolfe, L. K., Island, D. P., and Liddle, G. W. A diurnal rhythm in plasma renin activity in man. *J. Clin. Invest.* **45**:1587, 1966.
9. Brown, J. J., Davies, D. L., Lever, A. F., and Robertson, J. I. S. Influence of sodium loading and sodium depletion on plasma renin in man. *Lancet* **2**:278, 1963.

10. McKenzie, J. K., Ryan, J. W., and Lee, M. R. Effect of laparotomy on plasma renin activity in the rabbit. *Nature* **215**:542, 1967.
11. Vander, A. J. Control of renin release. *Physiol. Rev.* **47**:359, 1967.
12. Mannick, J. A., Huvos, A., and Hollander, W. E. Post-hydralazine renin release in the diagnosis of renovascular hypertension. *Ann. Surg.* **170**:409, 1969.
13. Mohammed, S., Fasola, A. F., Privitera, P. J., Lipicky, R. J., Martz, B. L., and Gaffney, T. E. Effect of methyldopa on plasma renin activity in man. *Circ. Res.* **25**:543, 1969.
14. Strong, C. G., Hunt, J. C., Sheps, S. G., Tucker, R. M., and Bernatz, P. E. Renal venous renin activity: Enhancement of sensitivity of lateralization by sodium depletion *Am. J. Cardiol.* **27**:602, 1971.
15. Simmons, J. L., and Michelakis, A. M. Renovascular hypertension: The diagnostic value of renal vein renin ratios. *J. Urol.* **104**:497, 1970.
16. Kaufman, J. J., Lupu, A. N., Franklin, S., and Maxwell, M. H. Diagnostic and predicative value of renal vein renin activity in renovascular hypertension. *J. Urol.* **103**:702, 1970.
17. Gunnells, J. C., McGuffin, W. L., Jr., Johnsrude, I., and Robinson, R. R. Peripheral and renal venous plasma renin activity in hypertension. *Ann. Int. Med.* **71**:555, 1969.
18. Michelakis, A. M., and Simmons, J. Effect of posture on renal vein renin activity in hypertension: Its implications in the management of patients with renovascular hypertension. *J.A.M.A.* **208**:659, 1969.
19. Kaneko, Y., Ikeda, T., Takeda, T., and Ueda, H. Renin release during acute reduction of arterial pressure in normotensive subjects and patients with renovascular hypertension. *J. Clin. Invest.* **46**:705, 1967.
20. Gross, F., Schaechtelin, G., Brunner, H., and Peters, G. The role of the renin–angiotensin system in blood pressure regulation and kidney function. *Canad. Med. Assoc. J.* **90**:258, 1964.
21. Stamey, T. A. Some observations on the filtration fraction, on the transport of sodium and water in the ischemic kidney, and on the prognostic importance of R.P.F. to the contralateral kidney in renovascular hypertension. *In Ciba Foundation Symposium on Antihypertensive Therapy*, Springer-Verlag, Heidelberg, p. 555, 1966.
22. Fair, W. R., and Stamey, T. A. Differential renal function studies in segmental renal ischemia. *J.A.M.A.* **217**:790, 1971.
23. Fair, W. R. Difficulties in the evaluation of hypertension secondary to renal ischemia. *Urol. Internat.* **25**:353, 1970.
24. Stamey, T. A., and Pfau, A. Some functional, pathological, bacteriological, and chemotherapeutic characteristics of unilateral pyelonephritis in man (Part I). *Invest. Urol.* **1**:134, 1963.

Horseshoe Kidney: Discordance in Monozygotic Twins

Elliot Leiter*

It is generally assumed that a demonstrated congenital defect in one of a pair of identical twins will be present in the other twin as well. Genotypic identity, however, does not always mean phenotypic identity. Discordant abnormalities in identical twins have been sporadically reported in the literature. We have recently seen a pair of identical twins who demonstrated just such discordance. Horseshoe kidney was present in one twin but absent in the other. We have been unable to find any previous report in the literature of the discordant occurrence of horseshoe kidney in monozygotic twins.

CASE REPORTS

J. C. (MSH No. 318438), a 28-year-old white male, was first seen at Mount Sinai Hospital in April 1966 with hypertension and uremia. Intravenous urogram showed poorly functioning but normally placed kidneys (Fig. 1). Percutaneous left renal needle biopsy showed chronic glomerulonephritis. The patient was placed on chronic hemodialysis in March 1968. In April 1968, his identical twin brother, D. C. (MSH No. 710800), was admitted for evaluation as a potential renal transplant donor. Intravenous urogram demonstrated a horseshoe kidney (Fig. 2). The presence of a thick connecting lower pole isthmus was confirmed on angiography. The ureters, bladder, and external genitalia of both siblings were normal.

*Associate Professor of Urology, Mount Sinai School of Medicine, of the City University of New York, New York, N.Y.

151

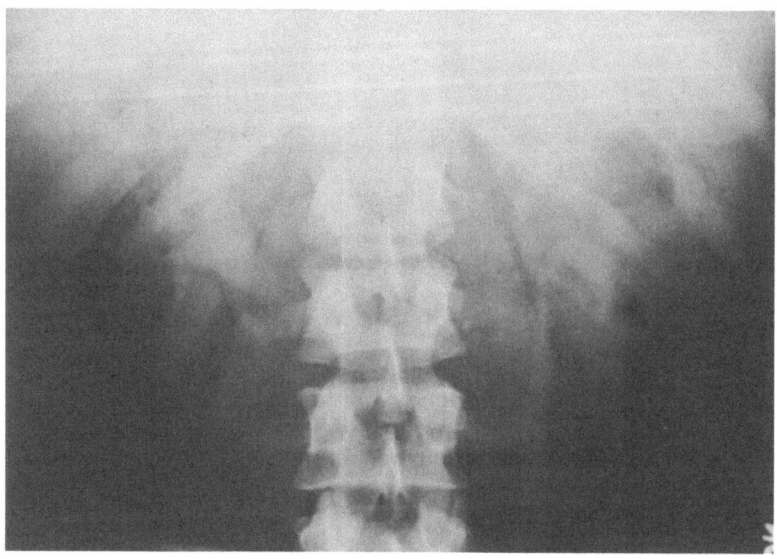

Fig. 1. Intravenous urogram of twin J. C. showing paired kidneys in normal position.

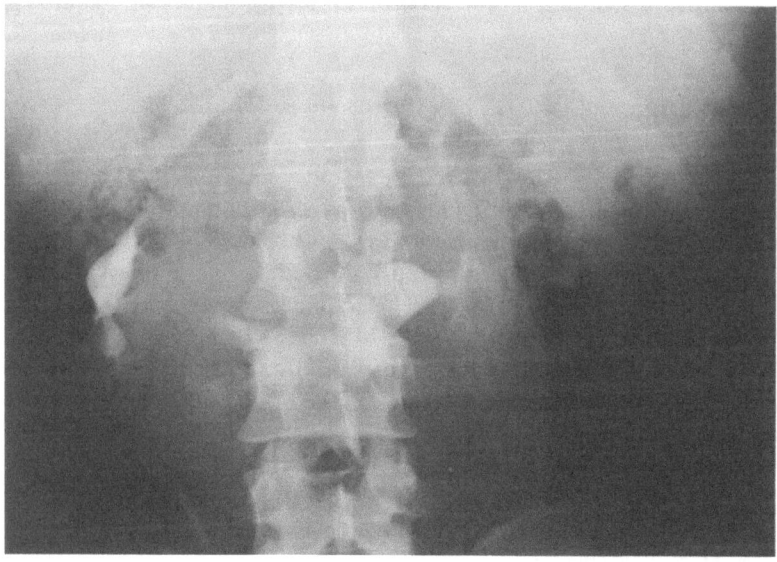

Fig. 2. Intravenous urogram of twin D. C. showing horseshoe kidney with very thick isthmus.

Red cell typing, white cell typing, and mixed lymphocyte culture were performed on both brothers. Identical red cell groups (B, Rh1, Rh2, DCe Pk, Kpb MNSs) as well as identicality at the HLA locus were demonstrated. There was no evidence of reactivity on mixed lymphocyte culture. Crossed skin grafts were performed. No rejection by either twin was demonstrated. J. C. subsequently underwent renal homotransplantation from a cadaver donor in September 1968. At the time of transplantation, left nephrectomy was performed. The kidney showed end-stage glomerulonephritis. D. C. remains well.

DISCUSSION

Discordant genitourinary defects in monozygotic twins have been reported only rarely. Reule and Ansell[1] presented five instances of discordance for urogenital defects in living identical twins. Monozygosity was substantiated by blood group comparison alone. Of the five reported cases, three involved fusional defects—one second-degree hypospadias, one bladder exstrophy, and one lumbar myelomeningocele with a neurogenic bladder. Four of the five reported pairs were males. Sorensen[2], again using identical red blood cell antigens as the criterion for monozygosity, described four pairs of twins in which there was discordant hypospadias in one member of each pair. In the few other reported cases of discordant genitourinary defects, the criteria for establishment of monozygosity have been much less strict[3-6]. We have been unable to find any reports in which monozygosity was established, beyond a doubt, by identicality of red and white cell antigens, mixed lymphocyte culture, and crossed skin grafts. Nor have we uncovered any previous description of a discordant fusional renal defect. In fact, Bridge[7] has reported horseshoe kidney occurring in two brothers presumed to be monozygotic twins.

Of interest is the fact that of the eight reported cases of discordance in which monozygosity is likely, all but one involved male twins, six were fusional defects, and five were patients with hypospadias. This apparent preponderance of male twins with discordant fusional defects has not to our knowledge been noted before.

Many described discordant defects have involved so-called lateral inversions. These may vary from complete situs inversus to mirror imaging of skin and hair patterns[8,9]. These discordant defects are felt to be related to the normal differences between the right and left sides of a single individual[10]. They seem more likely to occur when embryonic scission is relatively late and there is less chance for complete recovery of normal asymmetry.

The etiology of other discordant defects in identical twins is less clear. Intrauterine genetic mutations, cytoplasmic inheritance factors, pressure on one fetus by the placenta or the other fetus, as well as differences in placental blood flow and other environmental factors, have all been suggested. It is important to stress, however, that discordance does not unequivocally rule out heredity as an etiological factor in the observed anomaly. Gates[11] has suggested that unfavorable environmental conditions may lower the threshold for abnormal genes. Gruenwald and Mayberger[12], in discussing sirenoid malformations, note that "the pattern of defects found in late stages does not reflect the extent of the original abnormality in the very early embryo; it is most likely that the extent of the abnormality is influenced by mutual relations of the various primordia during their development." Trasler[13] has suggested that embryonic uterine location in rats may affect the expression of hereditary traits.

The previously noted report[7] of concordant horseshoe kidney in both members of a pair of twins as well as the common occurrence of other congenital anomalies in association with horseshoe kidney[14] lends credence to the possibility that the occurrence of horseshoe kidney may be related to specific intrauterine conditions favorable to the expression of an abnormal gene that is ordinarily of low penetrance.

SUMMARY AND CONCLUSIONS

A pair of identical twins, one with normally paired kidneys and the other with a horseshoe kidney, is described. Monozygosity was proven by identical red and white blood cell groups, mixed lymphocyte culture, and lack of rejection of crossed skin grafts.

Review of the literature failed to reveal any previous reported cases of discordant renal fusional defects in identical twins.

It is difficult to prove, solely on the basis of discordance in identical twins, whether horseshoe kidney and other renal fusional anomalies are genetically determined or not.

REFERENCES

1. Reule, G. R., and Ansell, J. S. Discordant occurrence of genitourinary defects in monozygotic twins. *J. Urol.* 97:1078–1081, 1967.
2. Sorensen, H. R. *Hypospadias with Special Reference to Aetiology,* Ejnar Munksgaard, Copenhagen, pp. 61 and 65, 1953.
3. Apert, M. E. Nanisme rénal et gémellité. *Bull. Soc. Med. Hop. Paris.* 1:232–235, 1934.
4. Guldberg, E. Verschiedengeschlechtige eineiige Zwillinge. *Acta Pathol. Microbiol. Scand. Suppl.* 37:197–223, 1938.
5. Morison, J. E. Congenital malformations in one of monozygotic twins. *Arch. Dis Child.* 24:214–218, 1949.
6. Hallgren, B., Larsson, H., and Rudhe, U. Nocturnal enuresis in twins. II. Urethrocystographic examinations. *Acta Pediat.* 50:117–126, 1961.
7. Bridge, R. A. C. Horseshoe kidneys in identical twins. *Brit. J. Urol.* 32:32–33, 1960.

8. Newman, H. H., and Quisenberry, W. B. One-egg twins with spina bifida and polydactyly. *J. Hered.* **35**:309–314, 1944.
9. Torgersen, J. Genic factors in visceral asymmetry and in the development and pathologic changes of lungs, heart and abdominal organs. *Arch. Pathol.* **47**:566–593, 1949.
10. Price, B. Primary biases in twin studies: A review of prenatal and natal difference-producing factors in monozygotic pairs. *Am. J. Hum. Genet.* **2**:293–352, 1950.
11. Gates, R. R. *Human Genetics*, Macmillan, New York, 1946.
12. Gruenwald, P., and Mayberger, H. W. Differences in abnormal development of monozygotic twins. *Arch. Pathol.* **70**:685–695, 1960.
13. Trasler, D. G. Influence of uterine site on occurrence of spontaneous cleft lip in mice. *Science* **132**:420–421, 1960.
14. Zondek, L. H., and Zondek, T. Horseshoe kidney and associated congenital malformations. *Urol. Internat.* **18**:347, 1964.

Renal Metabolism in Obstructive Uropathy

Horst K. A. Schirmer*

Through the encouragement and generosity of Dr. Willaim W. Scott, this investigation was made possible. His never-ending enthusiasm and inspiration brought problems encountered in the care of the sick to the Brady Research Laboratory—an investigator's haven created and supported by Dr. Scott's efforts. It is with great appreciation and thanks that I dedicate this paper to the Festschrift in honor of Dr. Scott's twenty-fifth anniversary as Professor of the Brady Urological Institute.

Many of our present concepts in obstructive uropathy are based on Hinman's observations with respect to hydronephrotic atrophy subsequent to complete obstruction of the flow of urine and the existence of a renal counterbalance where an anatomical and functional readjustment between the less injured or uninjured portion and the more injured portion in terms of performance takes place[1]. Together with Hepler, he introduced the concept of ischemia as possible cause for a hastening of dilatation and atrophy of the kidney with obstructed urine flow[2].

Previous experiments conducted in the Brady Research Laboratory on effects of ischemia and hypoxia upon renal metabolism indicated a shift in the Pasteur effect, with greater utilization of glucose and with lactic acid as intermediary end-product in renal cortical tissue[3-5].

*The James Buchanan Brady Urological Institute, The Johns Hopkins Hospital, Baltimore, Maryland.

157

In an effort to study the effects of acute and complete obstruction of the flow of urine upon renal metabolism, the following series of experiments were performed in the Brady Research Laboratory with the much appreciated and able assistance of Dr. Charles Tesar and coworkers.

Seemingly healthy adult mongrel dogs of both sexes were used in this study. Their left ureters were occluded in the terminal portion with a zero silk ligature under aseptic conditions. The contralateral intact kidney was biopsied and the tissue was processed for metabolic measurements. Fourteen days later, a biopsy was taken from the midportion of the hydronephrotic kidney cortex and the ligature around the distal ureter was released. Seven days following the release of the ureteral ligature, a second biopsy was taken from the hydronephrotic cortex, and at the same time the ureter of the up-to-this-point intact contralateral kidney was obstructed by silk ligature in its distal portion. Seven days following the occlusion of the previously intact ureter, biopsies were taken from both kidneys for final metabolic measurements.

Slices of tissue were prepared immediately from the biopsy specimens. The thickness of slices approximated 0.4 mm. After weighing, the slices were suspended in isotonic solutions buffered at pH 7.4 and contained within the main chambers of Warburg reaction vessels[6]. The vessels were mounted on manometers and immersed in the thermobath with the temperature at 37 C. The shaker speed was 120 cycle/min in semicircular fashion. Following perfusion of the vessels with 100% oxygen for the aerobic phase and 95% argon and 5% carbon dioxide for the anaerobic phase, and equilibration, pressures were recorded on the manometers at 10-min intervals for 60 min. Oxygen consumption by the tissue slices was determined in Krebs–Ringer phosphate solution which contained glucose[6]. The tissue wet weight: dry weight ratio was established by drying the tissue slices to constant weight. Metabolic quotients $Q_{O_2}^{O_2}$* and $Q_{CO_2}^{argon}$† were calculated on the basis of gas pressure changes per tissue weight per time.

Oxygen consumption of the intact canine renal cortex at the beginning of the experiment was 9.1 μl per milligram tissue dry weight per hour. When rendered anaerobic *in vitro*, the same amount of tissue produced 1.4 μl of lactic acid per hour. Fourteen days of ureteral occlusion accomplished the development of hydronephrosis with a reduction in oxygen consumption to one third of normal. Seven days following the release of the ipsilateral

---

*$Q_{O_2}^{O_2}$ is an expression for tissue respiration in terms of oxygen consumption and is defined as microliters of oxygen consumed per milligram dry weight of tissue per hour.

†$Q_{CO_2}^{argon}$ is an expression of anaerobic glycolysis in terms of carbon dioxide displacement on a mole-for-mole basis by lactic acid produced and is defined as microliters of carbon dioxide displaced from a Krebs–Ringer bicarbonate medium per milligram dry weight of tissue per hour.

ureteral obstruction, oxygen consumption increased above that determined at 14 days of obstruction. Oxygen consumption approached normal about 14 days following the release of ipsilateral ureteral obstruction and 7 days after obstruction of the contralateral ureter.

At 14 days of ureteral occlusion, anaerobic lactic acid formation in atrophic renal cortex was increased to four times that of normal. Seven days after the removal of the obstruction, glycolysis decreased to twice normal and was found to be within normal range 14 days after the release of the obstruction to the ipsilateral ureter, while the contralateral ureter was occluded for 7 days.

All six dogs survived the repetitive operative procedures, and no significant complications were encountered after ligation of the ureters, biopsy of the kidneys, or release of the ureteral occlusion.

The quotients for tissue respiration, $Q_{O_2}^{O_2}$, and anaerobic glycolysis, $Q_{CO_2}^{argon}$, are shown in Table. 1.

Complete ureteral occlusion by ligature thus induces the development of hydronephrotic parenchymal atrophy. The atrophic changes appear to closely parallel the metabolic development seen with ischemic hypoxia in renal cortical tissue, as oxygen consumption markedly decreases while its ability to produce lactic acid anaerobically increases to several times above normal. Such metabolic derangement is known as reversal of the Pasteur effect, with glucose as the preferred substrate and lactic acid as the intermediary end-product. Hinman and Hepler[2] considered ischemia to play an important role in the development of prenchymal atrophy. In their experiments they were able to observe that the reduction of arterial or venous blood flow in a kidney with obstructed urine flow effected a hastening of the development of parenchymal atrophy.

Whatever relationship to cause or effect the alterations in renal metabolism might have, they apparently closely follow alterations in renal function. Thus, a kidney with its urine flow completely obstructed for 14 day can recover to the state where in the presence of delayed occlusion of the

Table 1. Metabolism of Canine Renal Cortex Following Release of
Complete Ureteral Occlusion with Occluded Contralateral Ureter

	Normal	Ureteral occlusion (14 days)	7 days after release of occlusion	14 days after release of occlusion with ligature of contra- lateral ureter (7days)
$Q_{O_2}^{O_2}$	9.1	2.8	6.6	8.0
$Q_{CO_2}^{argon}$	1.4	5.4	2.4	1.1

contralateral ureter, it is capable of sustaining the life of its host. What role the status of the contralateral kidney plays in terms of degree of recovery can be appreciated by the examination of tissue respiration and glycolysis. Respiration and anaerobic glycolysis of atrophic renal cortical tissue in a recovery phase of 14 days following the release of ureteral occlusion can only approximate normal when the contralateral ureter is occluded.

Normalization of renal metabolism in a kidney recovering from hydronephrotic atrophy is therefore related to the status of its counterpart and is coupled with recovery of the oxidative tissue metabolism.

REFERENCES

1. Hinman, F. *The Principles and Practice of Urology,* W. B. Saunders Co., Philadelphia and London, pp. 487–527, 1935.
2. Hinman, F., and Hepler, A. Experimental hydronephrosis. The effect of ligature of one branch of the renal artery on its rate of development. *Arch. Surg.* **12**:830, 1926.
3. Schirmer, H. K. A. Renal metabolism in experimental hydronephrosis. *Invest. Urol.* **2**:598, 1965.
4. Schirmer, H. K. A., Murphy, G. P., Taft, J. L., and Scott, W. W. Renal metabolism with proximal or distal ureteral occlusion. *Surg. Gynec. Obstet.* **123**:539–543, 1966.
5. Schirmer, H. K. A., and Marshall, R. E. Metabolism of atrophic renal tissue following removal of complete ureteral obstruction. *J. Urol.* **100**:596, 1968.
6. Umbreit, W. W., Burris, R. H., and Stauffer, T. F. *Manometric Techniques,* Burgess Publishing Co., Minneapolis, p. 28, 1957.

The Nucleosides of Human Urine*

Arnold Mittelman

The most common product of the catabolism of nucleic acids is uric acid. Among its precursors are the purine nucleosides adenosine and guanosine present in deoxyribonucleic acid (DNA) and in ribonucleic acid (RNA). The general outline of the metabolic pathway is illustrated in Fig. 1. The importance of uric acid in a number of neoplastic and non-neoplastic disease states is well known. Our primary concern has been the identification of other nucleic acid metabolites that appear in human urine. Study of their origin, metabolic vicissitudes, and biological significance has been a major activity in our laboratory.

There are a number of species of human and generally mammalian nucleic acids that have been clearly identified during the past 10 years. These compounds are listed in Table 1. The composition of mammalian DNA is incompletely understood, but the bulk of this macromolecule is composed of four nucleosides (Fig. 2) with only a very small number of modified nucleosides such as 6-methylaminopurine deoxyriboside. Human ribonucleic acid, on the other hand, has a demonstrated complexity of species and structure that is the source of much current research. Ribosomal RNA consists of at least three identifiable species, two of which, 28s and 18s RNA, contain a small but measurable quantity of modified nucleosides[1,2]. 5s RNA, a small ribosomal unit, contains no modified nucleosides[3]. The postulated "messenger RNA" also seems devoid of unusual nucleosides and consists

*Supported by Grant CA-10835 and Grant RR-262 from the General Clinical Research Centers Program of the Division of Research Resources, National Institutes of Health, located at Roswell Park Memorial Institute and the State of New York Department of Health, Buffalo, New York.

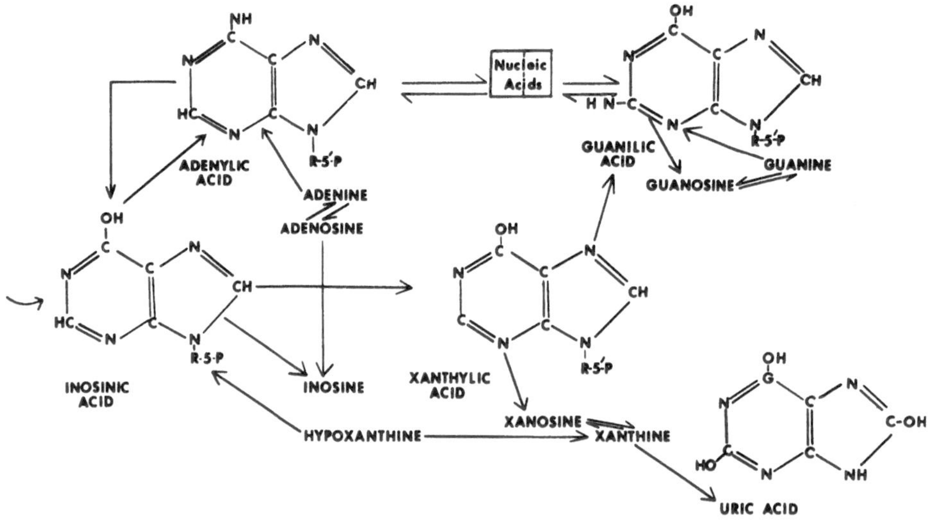

Fig. 1. This is the conventional metabolic pathway of all purines, regardless of origin. Uric acid in man is the end product of purine metabolism.

only of the four conventional ribonucleosides[4]. It is transfer RNA, the RNA that carries amino acids to the ribosome–messenger complex and forms the growing polypeptide chain, that contains many modified nucleosides[5,6]. A number of these nucleosides are present only in transfer RNA (tRNA), while others are present *predominantly*[7] in tRNA. It is with the modified nucleosides of tRNA that this study deals.

THE NUCLEOSIDE CONTENT OF HUMAN tRNA

The splenectomy program at Roswell Park Memorial Institute has provided large quantities of human tissue—normal, hyperplastic, and neo-

Table 1. Types of Mammalian Nucleic Acids

Type	Location
A. Deoxyribonucleic acid	Nucleus and mitochondria
B. Ribonucleic acid	Nucleus and cytoplasm
1. "Messenger" RNA	
2. Ribosomal RNA	
a. 28s, 18s, and 5s RNA type	
3. Transfer RNA	
a. At least one tRNA molecule for each amino acid	

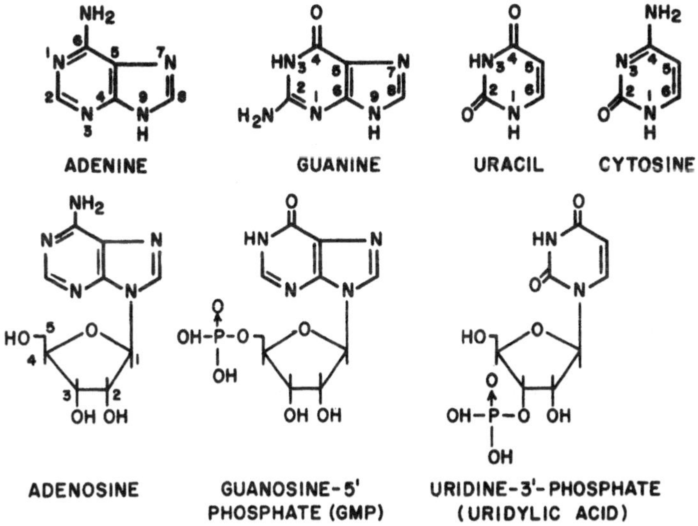

Fig. 2. Nonenclature of nucleic acid major components.

Table 2. Mole % Comparisons of Nucleosides of Different RNA Types

| Compound | Mole % | | |
	Human non-neoplastic	Human neoplastic	Yeast
Adenosine	18	22	17
Uridine	14	14	17
Guanosine	23	27	26
Cytidine	32	24	29
Pseudouridine	2.0	5.5	3.0
6-MAPR	0.6	1.6	
2'O-Me-uridine	0.8	1.6	
2'O-Me-cytidine	0.7	0.7	

plastic. The hyperplastic spleens come from patients with Felty's syndrome; the neoplastic are leukemic and lymphomatous spleens; the normal spleens are from partial gastrectomies for benign ulcer. Table 2 summarizes our findings. This list is by no means exhaustive. There are many more modified nucleosides present than we have tabulated. We present only those we have isolated and identified by conventional gravimetric and ultraviolet spectroscopy.

There are two nucleosides that are of particular interest to us. One of these is pseudouridine; the other is a more complex compound called

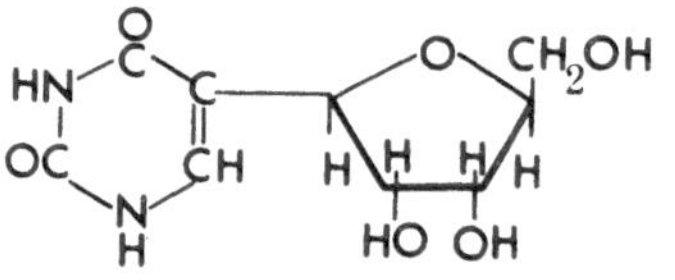

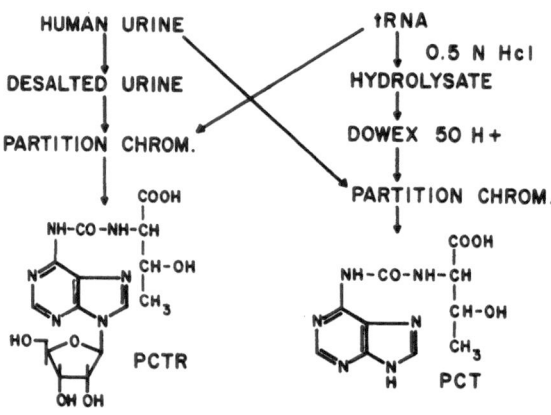

Fig. 3a. Pseudouridine. This unusual nucleoside demonstrates the carbon-to-carbon linkage of the uracil base to the pentose sugar via carbon-5 of the uracil skeleton.

N-(6-yl-carbamoylthreonine) riboside (PCTR) (Figs. 3a and 3b)(8). These are present exclusively in tRNA. Pseudouridine is present in Every tRNA that has been isolated from bacteria, yeast, or mammalian sources(9). PCTR is only present in those tRNAs whose codon begins with adenosine (first letter). The metabolic fate of these two nucleosides can yield considerable information concerning tRNA(10).

NUCLEOSIDES IN HUMAN URINE AND CALCULATION OF tRNA TURNOVER

We have found a number of nucleosides in human urine that are due to the breakdown of tRNA. These compounds are shown in Fig. 4. Pseudouridine and PCTR are among these urinary metabolites. Because of their particular chemical structure, their metabolic pathways have been clearly determined. Pseudouridine undergoes no metabolic change, and PCTR is

HUMAN URINE
DESALTED URINE
PARTITION CHROM.
tRNA
0.5 N HCl
HYDROLYSATE
DOWEX 50 H+
PARTITION CHROM.
PCTR
PCT
CHHEDA, et al BIOCHEMISTRY 8, 3278 (1969)
SCHWEIZER, et al BIOCHEMISTRY 8, 3283 (1969)
CHHEDA, LIFE SCIENCES AUG. (1969)

Fig. 3b. Sources and strueture of PCTR and PCT. PCTR is a unique nucleoside present exclusively in tRNA. It can be found in human urine at 0.04 mg/24 hr. This compound was isolated, identified, and synthesized at Roswell Park.

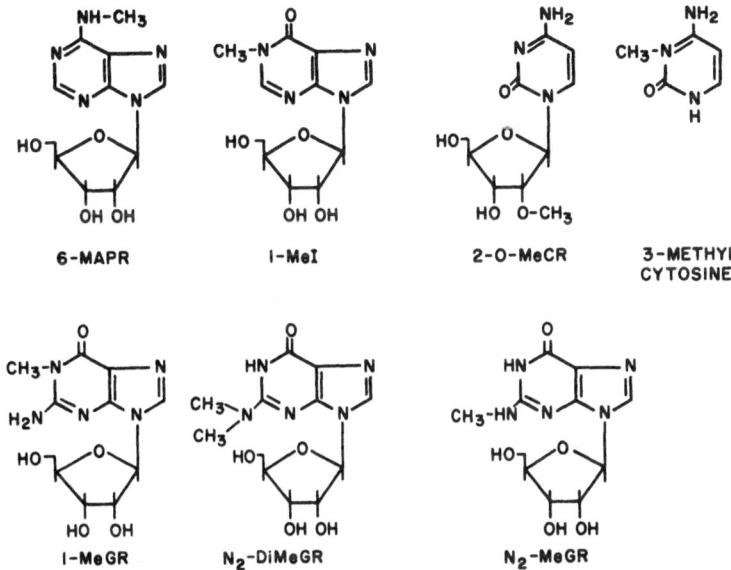

Fig. 4. Minor nucleosides isolated from human urine. These purine and pyrimidine nucleosides, all present in tRNA, have been isolated from human urine at Roswell Park. Improved isolation techniques demonstrate the predominance of the nucleoside over the base.

excreted 60–80% unchanged. The estimation of tRNA turnover in patients and normal subjects can be estimated from these data.

Given a controlled diet, pseudouridine levels vary little from day to day in a given individual. It is possible, therefore, to calculate the quantity of tRNA turnover in an individual under a variety of conditions. Such a calculation based on the urinary excretion of 40 mg and 3.5 mole % of pseudouridine is given below.

Amount of tRNA required to release 40 mg of pseudouridine

$$= \frac{\text{Urinary U(mg)}}{\text{mole \% } \times \text{ mol wt U}} \times \text{Av. mol wt nucleotide} \times 100$$

$$= \frac{40}{3.5 \times 244.2} \times 328 \times 100$$

$$= 1535 \text{ mg tRNA}$$

Normal subjects turn over approximately 1.5 g of tRNA daily. A practical application of this type of information may be found in our study of urinary pseudouridine and uric acid in surgical patients[11,12]. The normal response is indicated in Fig. 5. Similar data were obtained from patients with carcinoma of the prostate undergoing open and closed hypophysectomy.

BIOLOGICAL ACTIVITY OF URINARY NUCLEOSIDES

One of the earliest nucleosides assayed for biological activity was adenosine. The nucleoside when given intravenously caused hypotension and inhibited platelet aggregation. A number of modified adenosines such as PCTR, 1-methylinosine, N^6-methyladenosine may also have unique biological properties. All urinary constituents are being assayed for circulatory and platelet effects. Some of these appear to inhibit platelet aggregation without causing hypotension. The clinical usefulness of such substances in thromboembolic states would be considerable.

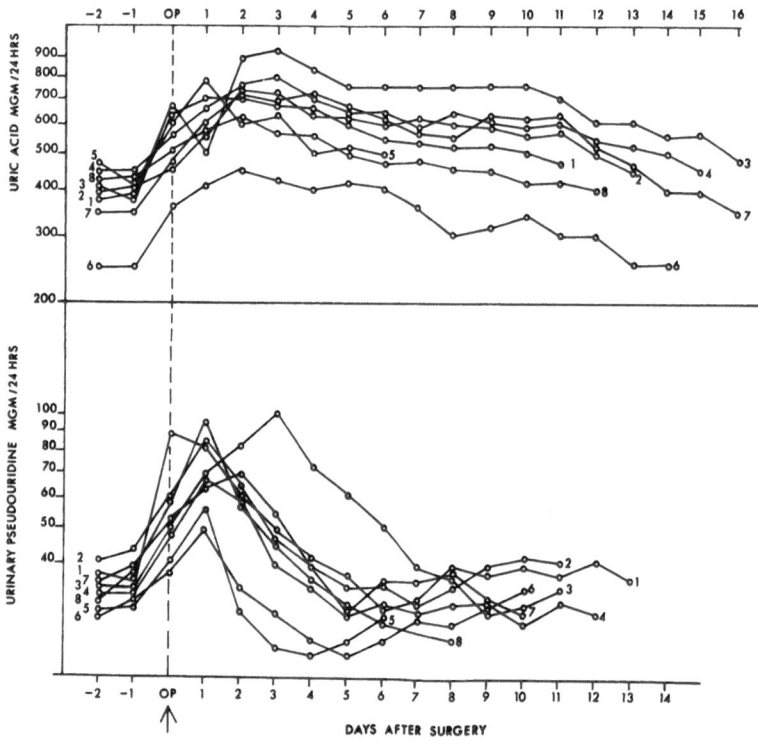

Fig. 5. Preoperative and postoperative uncomplicated cases. Levels of urinary pseudouridine and uric acid in the eight uncomplicated cases. The plots are semilogarithmic.

PCTR has been found to inhibit cell division of normal human lymphoblasts grown in tissue[13]. In addition, several analogues of PCTR have recently been shown to be cytokinins[14]. PCTR, 1-methylinosine, and isopentenyl adenosine (IPA) are all found in tRNA in a special location, i.e., adjacent to the anticodon. The modified nucleosides have been shown to be important for the binding of specific tRNAs to the messenger–ribosomal complex. If these modified nucleosides are altered or removed, then no attachment of the tRNA to the messenger–ribosomal complex can occur[15].

CONCLUSION

The picture that emerges is one of a dual function possessed by these modified nucleosides. As part of the macromolecule tRNA, these perform certain function. When the tRNA is metabolized, these nucleosides are released and circulate freely. Some are completely metabolized, such as IPA; others and their metabolites appear in the urine. Our work suggests that as free, circulating nucleosides, these substances exert a spectrum of biological activity. It is possible that they are part of a system of feedback control of macromolecular and protein synthesis.

The acceleration of nucleic acid metabolism, particularly tRNA metabolism, is a feature of surgical stress and infection, The magnitude of the stress is measured in the increased excretion of nucleic acid metabolites, i.e., uric acid and pseudouridine. We may speculate that some of the physiological reactions to stress, such as cardiovascular and coagulation changes, may be due in part to the breakdown products of tRNA, the modified nucleosides specifically, that we have found in human urine.

SUMMARY

We have isolated and measured a number of nucleosides in human urine. These arise as the result of the catabolism of transfer RNA (tRNA). Their appearance in the urine is increased by surgical stress. There is a correlation between the magnitude of the stress and the quantity of nucleosides found in urine. It is possible to calculate the turnover of human tRNA. These modified nucleosides may play a role in the regulation of protein synthesis and may, in part, be responsible for some of the physiological changes observed after surgical stress.

REFERENCES

1. Brown, G. M., and Attardi, G. *Biochem. Biophys. Res. Commun.* **20**:298, 1965.
2. Tamaoki, T., and Lane, G. B. *Biochemistry* **7**:3431, 1968.
3. Sanger, F., Brownlee, G., and Barrell, B. G. Proceedings of the Fourth Meeting, Federations of European Biochemical Societies, Oslo, July 1967.
4. Borek, E., and Srinivasan, P. R. *Ann. Rev. Biochem.* **35**:275, 1966.

5. Zachau, H. G. *Angew. Chem.* **8**:645, 1969.
6. Dunn, D. B., and Hall, R. In *Handbook of Chemistry,* Sober, H. A. (ed.), The Chemical Rubber Co., Cleveland, Ohio, p. G–3, 1968.
7. Starr, J. L., and Sello, B. H. *Phys. Rev.* **49**:623, 1969.
8. Schweizer, M. P., Chheda, G. B., Hall, R. H., Baczynskyj, L., and Biemann, K. *Biochemistry* **8**:3283, 1969.
9. Chheda, G. B., Hall, R. H., Magrath, D. L., Mozejko, J., Schweizer, M. P., Stasiuk, L., and Taylor, P. R. *Biochemistry* **8**:3278, 1969.
10. Chheda, G. B. *Life Sci.* **8**:979, Part II, 1969.
11. Schoonees, R., Mittelman, A., Chheda, G. B., and Murphy, G. P. *J. Surg. Oncol.* (in press).
12. Mittelman, A., Chheda, G. B., and Grace, J. T., Jr. *J. Surg. Res.* (in press).
13. Tritsch, G. L., Chheda, G. B., and Mittelman, A. Unpublished data.
14. Dyson, W. H., Chen, C. M., Alam, S. H., Hall, R. H., Hong, C. I., and Chheda, G. B. *Science* **170**:328, 1970.
15. Fittler, F., and Hall, R. H. *Biochem. Biophys. Res. Commun.* **25**:441, 1966.

Hypospadias: Experience with a One-Stage Repair (Hodgson Urethroplasty)

Rainer M. E. Engel*

For a long time I have been attracted, medically speaking, by the lower genitourinary tract; its numerous abnormalities and their embryological pathogenesis seem fascinating to me, and it was natural that I soon became intrigued by the potentials of hypospadias repairs. "Penile cripples," as Devine calls them, impressed upon me the need for a good one-stage repair.

Then, in the spring of 1968, Dr. W. W. Scott came back from a visit at Marquette University School of Medicine, where he had observed Norman Hodgson using a new one-stage repair. He was so enthused about this procedure and its relative freedom from complications that we soon did most of our hypospadias repairs with this method, as it allowed us, in one sitting, release of chordee and construction of a new distal urethra with the external meatus near or at the tip of the glans.

This one-stage urethroplasty can be performed in almost all patients with penile hypospadias, with or without chordee, if sufficient preputial skin is available.

METHOD

The method to be described is essentially that described by Hodgson for hypospadias occurring in the distal third of the penile shaft, with minor changes which we have made as we have gained experience.

*The James Buchanan Brady Urological Institute, The Johns Hopkins Hospital, Baltimore, Maryland.

After dilation of the hypospadiac meatus, the urine is diverted with a No. 14F balloon catheter introduced into the bladder through a perineal urethrostomy. It is held in place by inflation of the balloon and by a suture of silk or nylon placed through the edge of the skin incision and then tied around the catheter.

The incision in the deep preputial layer begins in a circumferential line just below the coronal sulcus. It is extended through the skin of the ventrum of the shaft to the point of beginning on the dorsal surface. The hypospadiac meatus is circumscribed. This is done by making a triangular incision whose base is at the coronal sulcus and whose long limbs meet in the midline just below the urethral meatus. Then all fibrous tissue causing chordee is excised down to the tunica albuginea of the corpora cavernosa and far enough laterally to completely release the chordee. The distal urethra is mobilized if necessary.

We then place three stay-sutures through the dorsal hood, rather than using skin hooks. These are placed at points where the deep and superficial preputial layers meet, two at each lateral margin and one in the midline. Parallel incisions are then made through the deep preputial layer (mucosal surface) of the hood. These extend from the base of this layer toward the junction of the deep and superficial (cutaneous surface) layers. This deep preputial tissue will become the new urethra. These incisions are through the cutis only and should avoid all blood vessels. The width of this flap should be about 2 cm, wider in older children, and the length adjusted to bridge the gap between the circumscribed hypospadiac meatus and the tip of the glans penis. The redundant deep preputial layer lateral to the flap is then excised. The dorsal skin of the penis is then separated by blunt dissection from the shaft with scissors for two thirds of the length of the penis.

Next, a buttonhole is made through the skin of the dorsum of the penis, permitting the glans and distal shaft to be pulled through this buttonhole. This incision is in the midline with lateral relaxing incisions made, if necessary, after the pull-through. A stay-suture through the tip of the glans helps in this maneuver.

A tube is fashioned from the deep preputial flap. This is done around a Silastic stent. The sutures used are interrupted 6–0 chromic catgut. They are carefully placed through the subcutaneous tissue just beneath the lateral margins of the flap but not through it.

The new urethra is now joined to the circumscribed urethral meatus, the latter trimmed to size. The same suture material is used as in rolling the flap. The posterior surface is sutured first after the flap has been turned over. This maneuver brings the suture line of the new urethra into the groove between the corpora cavernosa, away from the ventral skin covering and thus reducing the chance of a fistula.

Small wedge incisions are then made into the penile glans. These run about 2 mm parallel to the midline of the urethral groove, bilaterally. The external meatus of the new urethra is sewn to the medial margin of these lateral incisions.

The penile skin is closed with interrupted 5- to 6–0 nylon sutures after the redundant lateral "dog-ears" have been resected. At the new meatus, the skin is also sewn to the lateral margins of the wedge incisions in the penile glans. The holding suture through the tip of the glans is used to tie in the urethral stent and is then sewn into the anterior abdominal wall. Adequate hemostasis is most important throughout the procedure. Sponges soaked in a 1:100,000 solution of epinephrine and applied to the wound aid in hemostasis, and fine bleeding-points are then coagulated with the cauterizing needle. At the close of the procedure, we cover the wound with Adaptic and apply a very light protective dressing. We believe that a pressure dressing should *not* be used, as complications frequently seen following urethroplasty may be due in part to compression of the vascular supply by these dressings. Bedrest is compulsory for the first few days.

Sutures and urethral stent are removed on the tenth postoperative day under light general anesthesia; the balloon retention catheter is removed the following day.

RESULTS

Between May 1969 and January 1971, we performed 24 urethroplasties using the method described. Three of these patients had previously undergone partial circumcision of their dorsal hoods. The results of these repairs have been very satisfactory; complications were encountered in the early period, but the last ten patients have been complication free.

No patient developed a wound breakdown or infection. One patient developed a small fistula at the site of the anastomosis of the hypospadiac meatus to the new urethra and eventually formed a stenosing scar in this area. During the next year, it was necessary to perform a two-stage Johanson urethroplasty on him; presently, this patient is doing very well.

A small fistula at the anastomosis site occurred in another patient and was closed surgically. No stenosis of the newly formed urethra occurred, but a mild stenosis at the juncture of old to new urethra was seen in two other patients. One of these had a meatal stenosis, too. These stenoses were dilated easily, under sedation or general anesthesia, and have not required further instrumentation. Two further patients with meatal stenosis were seen; one has been dilated satisfactorily, while the other underwent a meatotomy. Both have done well.

SUMMARY

Twenty-four patients underwent a Hodgson urethroplasty for hypospadias with chordee. Five patients developed stenosis; of these, two had meatal stenosis, two others stenosis at the anastomosis site of urethra to new urethra, and one stenosis in both areas. Two patients developed a fistual at the anastomosis site, and one of these is also a patient who had a stenosis at the anastomosis site. Thus, a total of six patients developed complications, and three of these had to be repaired surgically.

The Hodgson one-stage urethroplasty is the urethroplasty of choice for a selected number of patients. The complications are minimal, and the results very satisfactory.

Rationale for the Use of Nonabsorbable Antibiotics in the Treatment of Urinary Infections: Follow-Up Report

Herbert Schwartz*

Dr. W. W. Scott has recognized, these last several years, my keen interest in the causes and management of urinary tract infections. He has continuously encouraged my investigations, provided laboratory space and research tools, been constantly available for consultation and advice. In addition, as my studies began to bear fruit and I was ready for clinical investigations, he was the first to make available his patients for study and treatment. As a result of these efforts, a group of patients has been treated for a period of up to $2\frac{1}{2}$ year with various forms of nonabsorbable sulfonamides, in particular, Neothalidine followed by Sulfathalidine. The following paper is a report concerning the treatment of 36 such patients.

Gram-negative bacteria, particularly those that comprise the loosely termed coliform group, are responsible for 70–80 % of urinary infections[1-4]. This is true for patients in a domiciliary as well as a hospital practice[5,6], through the frequency of infecting organisms varies considerably between these two groups.

In hospitalized patients, particularly those with an associated urological problem, the infecting organisms usually encountered are *Klebsiella aerogenes* and *Escherichia coli* with *Proteus* species and *Pseudomonas* species being found to a lesser degree[4,7].

*The James Buchanan Brady Urological Institute. The Johns Hopkins Hospital, Baltimore, Maryland.

It has been my clinical impression as well as that of other investigators that many patients with recurrent urinary infections have complained of gaseous distention, chronic constipation, diarrhea, and other similar gastrointestinal symptoms closely preceding an attack[8-10].

We have previously reported, as part of continuous studies now underway regarding the etiology and treatment of urinary infections, the following:

1. *E. coli,* genetically identified with specific antisera to its somatic (O) antigens[4,11] and labeled with tritiated thymidine, when inoculated intramucosally into the sigmoid colon of dogs, did invade the parenchyma of a previously damaged kidney and was recovered by tissue cultures of the kidney and demonstrated by autoradiographs[12].

2. There is a significant correlation between organisms isolated simultaneously from the urine and stool of patients suffering from urinary infections[4,7].

3. Patients with an *E. coli* bacteriuria had a serotypically identical mate in a simultaneously cultured stool specimen in almost every instance, O serotype 0119 being the most common[7].

These premises support the view that the organisms of the gastrointestinal tract play a significant role in the perpetuation of an individual's urinary infection regardless of the means by which they may reach the urinary tract, i.e., from the blood or lymph or by direct perineal contamination and ascension.

The majority of acute infections of the lower or upper tract usually can be controlled initially by one or more of the available systemically active antibiotics, provided no major organic abnormality exists. However, infection often recurs at various intervals once therapy is discontinued. Calculus or stasis, for example, will perpetuate an infection regardless of the use of the most efficient means of chemotherapy. In some individuals without any demonstrable abnormality, infection will persist in a chronic state. Such chronic or frequently recurring infections generally result in slowly progressive damage to the kidneys and, furthermore, may lead to the ultimately debilitating "chronic" pyelonephritis. It is most important, therefore, that use be made of every available means to accomplish complete and permanent eradication of urinary infections of this type.

In the case of coliform infections, the normal flora of the intestinal tract constitutes a permanent massive reservoir of the offending organisms. Thus, patients with a matching organism in the stool similar to that causing the urinary infection could be treated by attacking the reservoir. Furthermore, if this reservoir could be controlled, indeed the episodes of recurrence and chronicity might be eliminated.

Thus, an antibacterial agent that exhibits little or no absorption from the gastrointestinal tract, that exerts its effect upon the bacterial flora of the large bowel, and that has minimal to no toxic effects if absorbed would be desirable in these cases. Credit must go to Poth([8,13]) and Everett([9,10]) for suggesting, back in the early 1940s while working with succinylsulfathiazole and phthalylsulfathiazole, that this might be a legitimate form of treatment.

These relatively nonabsorbable sulfonamides have been in use for years in the treatment of bacillary dysentery, diarrhea, and ulcerative colitis and as bowel preparations before gastrointestinal surgery. Succinylsulfathiazole and phthalylsulfathiazole have withstood the test of time in the above spheres of therapy and are minimally absorbed (95 % or more being excreted in the feces), minimally toxic, and effective against the coliforms, particularly *E. coli*([14]).

This report will deal with the effects of these relatively nonabsorbable sulfonamides in the long-term treatment of patients with recurrent urinary infections, the rationale being that suppression of bacteria in the colon may reduce the transit of bacteria to the urinary tract and allow the host's immunological response and normal defense mechanism to rid the urinary tract of invading bacteria.

Thirty-six patients were evaluated.

METHODS

The patients were selected because of (a) a history of persistent and recurrent urinary infections; (b) urinary infection present; (c) however, no definite predisposing anatomical abnormality as determined by intravenous pyelography, voiding cinecystourethrography, and cystoscopy where applicable and at the discretion of the examiner; (d) matching organisms in the urine and feces.

Urine was obtained, either as a clean-catch voided midstream specimen or directly from an indwelling urethral catheter, and streaked on blood agar (Baltimore Biological Laboratories) with a special loop that contains an inoculum of 0.01 ml. Both plates were incubated aerobically for 24 hr at 37 C.

Stool specimens were obtained by inserting a sterile swab into the rectal ampulla and then inoculating a small area of phenyl ethyl alcohol agar, deoxycholate agar, and *Salmonella–Shigella* agar (Baltimore Biological Laboratories). A small sample was placed on selenite-F enrichment broth (Baltimore Biological Laboratories). The media were then incubated for 12–18 hr at 37 C. When identification of the colonies was uncertain, further biochemical tests were performed according to the flow sheets in the clinical microbiology laboratory manual.

Where the infecting organism was *E. coli*, it was serotypically identified using a modification of the method described by Ewing([11]), and a match was sought in the rectal swab.

Table 1. Thirty-six Patients Receiving Long-Term Phthalylsulfathiazole Therapy

Infecting organism	Completed 2 years without infection	Treatment failures[a]
Escherichia coli	23	7
Klebsiella sp.	0	2
Staphylococcus epidermis	3	0
Proteus sp.	1	0
Pseudomonas sp.	0	0
	27	9

[a] Seven have an organic and/or functional abnormality of the GU tract.

Simultaneous urine and stool cultures were obtained at 3, 7, 14, 21, and 28 days and then at monthly intervals thereafter.

Urine cultures were considered significant when the colony count on two successive determinations was greater than 10^5 per milliliter regardless of symptoms, or greater than 10^4 per milliliter on successive determinations associated with related symptoms. A cure was defined as a negative culture on subsequent determinations or less than 10^4 associated with no urinary symptoms.

Upon each visit, the patient had blood drawn to determine any changes in the hematocrit, white blood cell count, serum Na, K, Cl, CO_2, bilirubin, and SGPT.

The treatment schedule was as follows: Four weeks on medications, interrupted by a 2-week rest period, to be continued for 1 year. Medications were Neothalidine, 1 tablespoon (15 ml) q.i.d. for 12 doses, to be followed by phthalylsulfathiazole, 1 g q.i.d.; menadione, 5 mg q.i.d.; multivitamin complex (with thiamine), 1 capsule q. am. Menadione and multivitamin (with thiamine) preparations were used to replace what is ordinarily produced by the intestinal flora.

RESULTS

Each patient had a matching organism in the feces. Thirty-six patients are being evaluated, and 27 have exceeded the 24-month treatment period without becoming reinfected and are currently being observed for recurrence. One patient, after 18 months (6 months off therapy) did develop an infection with Proteus mirabilis, the same genus and species causing the original infection. Nine patients did not respond to the treatment; seven of these were eventually shown to have an associated organic and/or functional abnormality of the urinary tract; seven individuals had E. coli infections, and two had Klebsiella infections. Table 1 indicates the urinary pathogens isolated in these patients.

Figures 1 and 2, respectively, represent graphically how the urine and feces were monitored in a representative patient "cured" after a 12-month course of suppressive therapy. The urine culture was negative on the third day (after the 12 doses of Neothalidine) and remained so for the entire 12 months. Note that with this treatment schedule the *E. coli* in the feces was never eradicated. However, the growths of *E. coli* leveled off to a countable range between 10^4 to 10^5 colonies per milliliter. This is certainly a sharp decrease considering the fact that one is dealing with bulk *E. coli* in faces.

There have been to significant alterations in the hematocrit, WBC, serum K, Na, Cl, CO_2, SGPT, or bilirubin.

One group of facts that deserves particular emphasis is that there have been *no* monilial or staphylococcal superinfections with this regimen. In cases where individuals were previously constipated, bowel movements became soft and more frequent. Several individuals, during their initial suppression of bowel infection with the Neothalidine, did develop mild abdominal cramps associated with loose bowel movements; however, these symptoms subsided rapidly upon completing the Neothalidine (neomycin and phthalylsulfathiazole) course and starting the phthalylsulfathiazole.

DISCUSSION AND CONCLUSIONS

It is recognized that the philosophy of suppression of a bacterial reservoir as a form of treatment or prophylaxis is not new. It has been effective

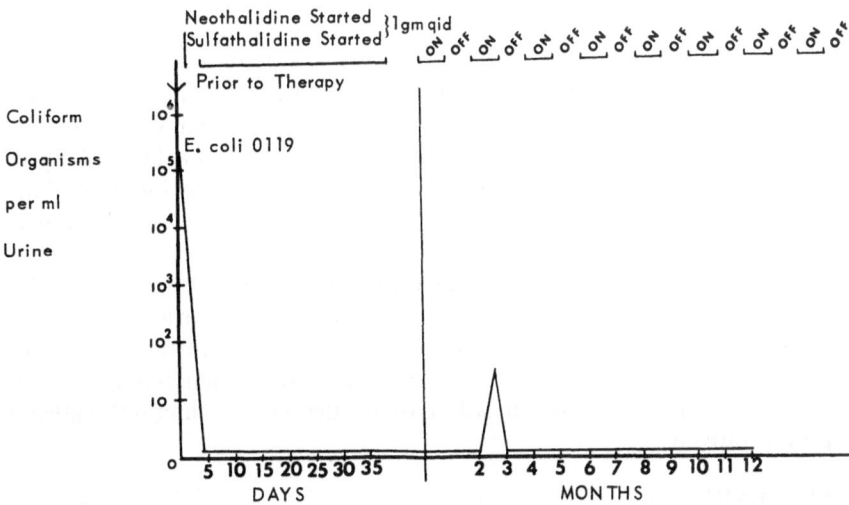

Fig. 1. Record of *E. coli* in urine. Note the rapid disappearance of *E. coli* bacteriuria after institution of Neothalidine and maintenance of suppression with course of phthalylsulfathiazole (1 g q.i.d.).

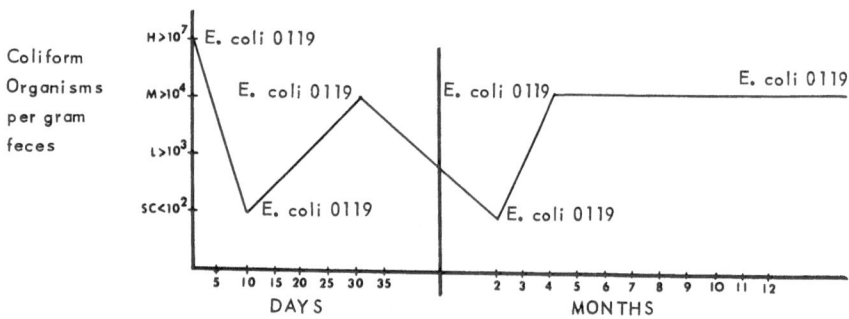

Fig. 2. Record of *E. coli* in feces. Note the rapid suppression at first of the fecal reservoir of *E. coli*. The organism is never eradicated from the gut but rather levels off at a count of 10^5 or less, which is significantly decreased for a gram of feces.

in eradicating or controlling rheumatic fever, tuberculosis, leprosy, and acne.

The control of symptomatic recurrent bacteriuria with relatively non-absorbable intestinal sulfonamides may eventually prove to be effective in the treatment of urinary infections. They now appear to be effective particularly in females, especially against *E. coli,* and particularly in individuals who have no demonstrable functional or anatomical abnormality of the urinary tract. Future studies should evaluate their use in children, particularly young girls, pregnant women, and patients in general in whom a chronic or recurrent bacteriuria may lead to permanent renal damage.

How did suppression of the bacterial reservoir in the gut allow for a clearing of the bacteriuria? It is possible that the perineal contamination in females was averted and ascending infection was prevented and/or that spread via the bloodstream and lymphatics from the gut was controlled. A relatively normal urinary tract may overcome infection by evoking the host's natural defense mechanisms (phagocytes, immunoglobulins, fluids, pH, osmolarity) or localized defense mechanisms located in the urinary tract.

Patient evaluations suggest that early studies should begin with evaluation of individuals with relatively normal urinary tracts, particularly females. Subsequent studies are evaluating the use of this mode of therapy in children, pregnant women, and adult males, particularly those undergoing prostatic or bladder operations which will require the use of urethral catheters postoperatively.

SUMMARY

A clinical evaluation of phthalylsulfathiazole in the treatment and prophylaxis of recurrent urinary infections is presented as part of a continuous study underway to determine the etiology and treatment of urinary infections. It appears that long-term treatment is effective in controlling recurrences. Individuals, particularly females, with apparently normal urinary tracts infected with *E. coli* are particularly responsive to this form of therapy. It may have its best use as a prophylactic agent in individuals with chronic or recurrent bacteriuria in whom the possibility of permanent and progressive renal damage is real.

REFERENCES

1. Campbell, M. F. *Urology,* W. B. Saunders Company, Philadelphia, Vol. 1, pp. 381–405, 1963.
2. Beeson, P. B. Factors in the pathogenesis of pyelonephritis. *Yale J. Biol. Med.* **28**:81–104, 1955.
3. Bush, I. M., Orkin, L. A., and Winter, J. An eleven year study of urinary bacterial cultures in a total in-patient hospital population. *J. Urol.* **94**:168–171, 1965.
4. Schwarz, H., Schirmer, H., Ehlers, B., and Post, B. Urinary tract infections: Correlation between organisms obtained simultaneously from the urine and feces of patients with bacteriuria and pyuria. *J. Urol.* **101**:756–767, 1969.
5. O'Grady, F., and Brumfitt, W. *Urinary Tract Infection,* Oxford University Press, London, pp. 68–79, 1968.
6. Kunin, C. M., Deutscher, R., and Paquin A. Urinary tract infection in school children: An epidemiological, clinical, and laboratory study. *Medicine* **43**:91–130, 1964.
7. Schwarz, H., Schirmer, H., Post, B., and Ehlers, B. Correlation of *Escherichia coil* occurring simultaneously in the urine and stool of patients with clinically significant bacteriuria: Serotyping with group-specific O antisera. *J. Urol.* **101**:379–382, 1969.
8. Poth, E. J., and Ross, C. A. The clinical use of phthalylsulfathiazole. *J. Lab. Clin. Med.* **29**:785–808, 1944.
9. Everett, H. S., Vosberg, G. A., and Davis, J. M. The treatment of urinary infections with sulfathalidine (phthalylsulfathiazole). *J. Urol.* **59**:83–91, 1948.
10. Everett, H. S., Scott, R. B., and Steptoe, P. P. The treatment of urinary infections with sulfasuxidine (succinylsulfathiazole). *Am. J. Obstet. Gynec.* **49**:114–127, 1945.
11. Ewing, W. H. *Isolation and Identification of E. coli Serotypes Associated with Diarrheal Diseases,* CDC Laboratory Manual, U.S. Dept. Health, Education and Welfare, Public Health Service, Communicable Disease Center, Laboratory Branch, Atlanta, Georgia, p. 10, 1963.
12. Schwarz, H. Renal invasion by *E. coli* via mucosal lesion of the sigmoid colon: A demonstration utilizing methods of autoradiography and group-specific serologic typing. *Invest. Urol.* **6**:98–113, 1968.
13. Poth, E. J. Sulfasuxidine and sulfathalidine. *Texas Rep. Biol. Med.* **4**:68–102, 1946.
14. Goodman, L. S., and Gillman, A. *The Pharmacological Basis of Therapeutics.* Macmillan, New York, pp. 1158–1160, 1965.

Vesicoureteral Reflux—Who Needs Ureteroneocystostomy?

James M. Holland*

Today the urologist treating a patient having recurrent urinary tract infections performs voiding cystourethrography almost as routinely as excretory pyelography (IVP) and cystoscopy. The high yield of vesicoureteral reflux, paraureteral diverticula, and bladder outlet obstruction has stimulated much creative work searching for cause and best treatment of these congential disorders.

Reflux had been demonstrated at the turn of this century, but its role in the cause of progressive renal damage was not generally appreciated until the 1950s([1]). Soon thereafter, the pathophysiology and effective surgical correction of reflux were well worked out, but opinion was often sharply divided on whether or not reflux was harmful enough to warrant antireflux surgery. Reflux often was shown to disappear after correction of distal obstruction, practice of multiple voiding techniques, and long-term drug treatment([2]). To those of us beginning our urological training around 1960 the disagreement among those advising reimplanting all refluxing ureters, or none, or whether or not to revise the bladder neck routinely was confusing at best. A prospective inquiry was needed to develop guidelines for rational treatment.

In the early 1960s here at Brady, Lowell King and Harry Mellins began to search for factors contributing to reflux and how to recognize when valvular damage had become severe enough to require surgical repair. Studies of bladder, ureteral, and urethral pressures were correlated with cineradiographic and cystoscopic appearance, then applied to management of the

*Department of Urology, Northwestern University School of Medicine, Chicago, Illinois.

patient. When Dr. King came to Children's Memorial Hospital in Chicago in 1963, he stimulated others in the Northwestern Urology Department who had agonized over the proper management of the refluxing ureter. Among them was John B. Graham, now my associate, whose patients are included in this study.

The purpose of this paper is to report our experience at Evanston Hospital, a Northwestern University Medical Center hospital which serves the suburbs just north of Chicago. Children comprise about one third of all our patients, who are referred primarily by physicians on the Evanston Hospital staff. Thus the patient population we see is a fair sample of that seen in a non–medical center practice.

PATIENT STUDY GROUP

Our series of patients shown to have vesicoureteral reflux now numbers 167, 11 of them adults (Table 1). Antireflux surgery was performed on 35 children and four adults. In all, 55 renal units were reimplanted, eight of them being duplicated ureters. Patients generally presented with a history of urinary infection with or without fever; enuresis was occasionally the only complaint. Of the 39 patients reimplanted, 35 had febrile urinary tract infections before age 5 and 16 showed pyelonephritic changes at the first work-up.

Voiding cystography was usually performed after infection was controlled. As image intensifiers improved and our radiologists became more experienced, we tended to rely more upon fluoroscopy and judicious spot films than continuous cine strips. These studies not only provided better diagnostic studies but also reduced radiation exposure. Except in the case of prostatic or distal urethral valves, we were not able to diagnose reliably meatal or distal urethral stenosis radiographically. An intravenous pyelogram was then done when refluxed contrast material had returned to the

Table 1

Operation		Female	Male	Total
Antireflux:	Children	31	4	35
	Adults	3	1	4
Nephrectomy:	Adults	4	0	4
None:	Adults	2	1	3
	Febrile UTI	71	2	73
	Afebrile UTI	33	6	39
	No UTI	3	6	9
		147	20	167

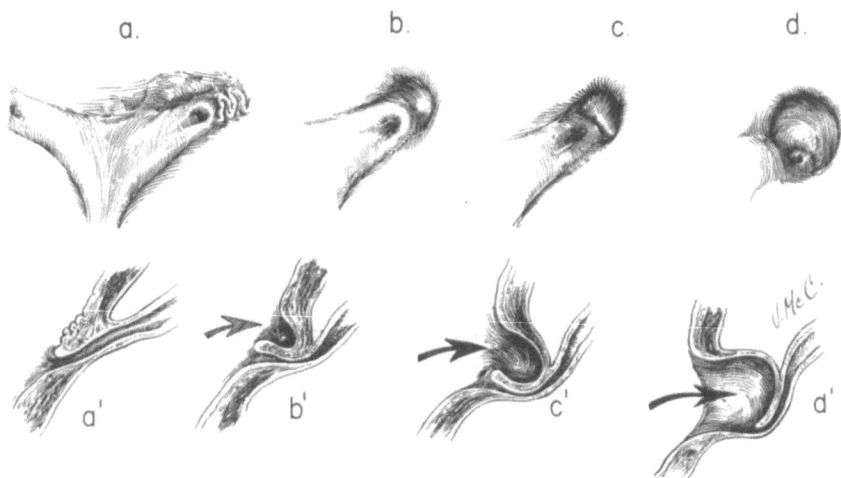

Fig. 1. Paraureteral diverticulum.

bladder. Ureteral dilatation and tortuosity seen on cystogram were often not apparent on the intravenous pyelogram.

Cystoscopy and urethral calibration were commonly done a day or two after radiographic studies. The urethra of females between 2 and 10 years should accept a 16 F Otis bougie without obstruction([3]). Adult females should accommodate a 24 F. Boys normally accept a 10 or 12 F bougie. Girls were routinely dilated to 24–28 F whether or not distal urethral stenosis was found; meatotomy was done for stenosis in both sexes. Boys were generally dilated only to 12 F as necessary for introduction of the infant cystoscope. We found bladder neck caliber difficult to judge reliably with the cystoscope; coarse trabeculation and significant residual urine were more certain signs of bladder outlet obstruction.

The ureteral orifices were inspected for appearance and location and were catheterized to measure length of the intramural ureter (the tunnel). A tunnel longer than 15 mm was called normal, although those 10–15 mm long generally did not allow reflux if properly buttressed and not involved in a diverticulum. Lax detrusor support of the intramural ureter was judged if it telescoped as the catheter was drawn in and out or by probing the roof of the tunnel with the catheter.

After removal of the ureteral catheter, the bladder was filled and anesthesia lightened until a spontaneous detrusor contraction ensued. Deficient intramural support could then be seen as shortening of the tunnel. Occasionally, dramatic herniation of a paraureteral diverticulum occurred as we watched, the ureteral orifice being pulled into the everted diverticulum (Fig. 1). Finding redundant rugose folds of bladder epithelium just superolateral to the ureteral orifice suggested presence of such a diverticulum. We believe each refluxing ureteral orifice should be inspected during a detrusor contraction.

Unless surgical intervention was clearly indicated, outlet obstruction was relieved, long-term antimicrobial agents were given, frequent and multiple voiding habits were encouraged, and high fluid intake and periodic urinalyses were advised. Repeat cystogram, intravenous pyelogram, and cystoscopy were done if infections recurred or if some damage was already present.

As a general rule, antireflux surgery was not necessary if the tunnel had reasonable length and support, while obstruction and infection were adequately treated. In such patients, inflammation of the valvular mechanism caused temporary regurgitation (Fig. 2). Thus even patients having relatively short tunnels could be spared surgery if bladder infections could be prevented. Long discussions with parents have been rewarded by more faithful follow-up and giving of drugs.

INDICATIONS FOR SURGICAL TREATMENT

Nearly all antireflux operations were performed to repair severe ureterovesical junction deformity in patients who had recurrent febrile infections and persisting reflux despite conservative treatment. In two patients, Y-V bladder neck plasty did not relieve reflux until ureteroneocystostomy was done. As our experience has increased, we have advised earlier reimplantation of refluxing ureters everting into a paraureteral diverticulum or having no intramural ureter (absent tunnel).

In four adults, renal damage was so advanced that nephrectomy was required.

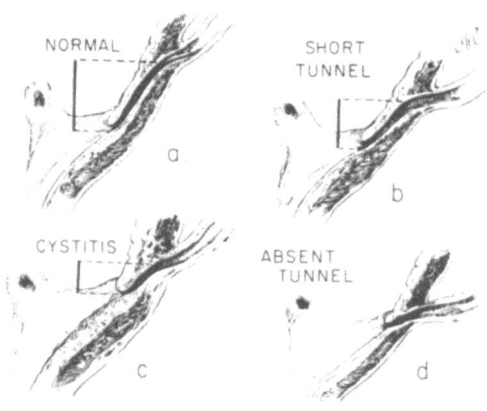

Fig. 2

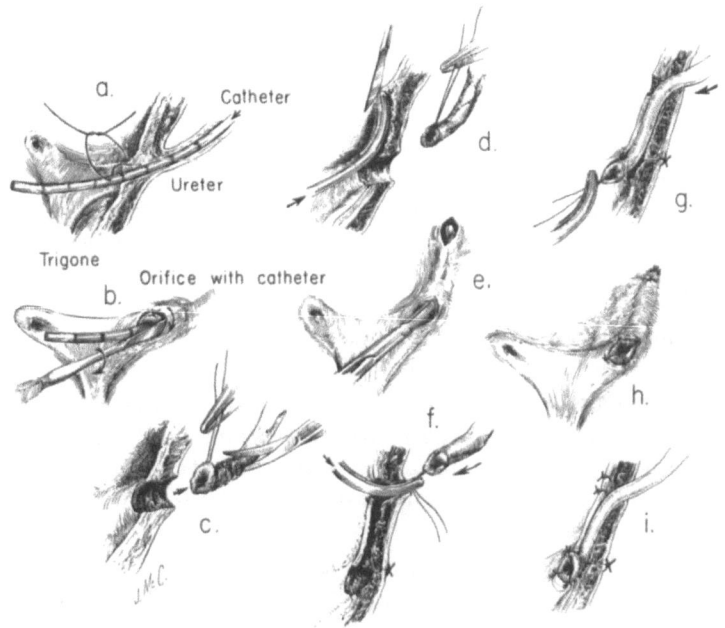

Fig. 3. Modified Politano reimplant.

SURGICAL PROCEDURE

In 37 of the 39 patients undergoing antireflux surgery (53 of the 55 ureteral units), a length of terminal ureter was placed in a new tunnel created between urothelium and detrusor muscle, as described by Politano and Leadbetter[4]. We altered this technique by mobilizing ureter for a short distance outside the bladder, taking care to preserve ureteral vessels (Fig. 3). This allowed us to divide bands or unnecessary arteries (obliterated hypogastric or uterine) which could obstruct the ureter. A generous new detrusor hiatus was made to prevent angulation. The new tunnel was made approximately 2–3 cm long. In about one third of the 53 ureters, the old intramural ureter was excised. No cuff or nipple was formed at the new ureterovesical junction. Stents were usually used and removed on the fifth day. T-tube ureterostomy was tried; each of the several times used, it was a disease state itself and a nuisance. In boys, all tubes are brought out suprapubically; in girls, they may be led through the urethra.

The ureters of eight operated-on units were duplicated. Pyeloureterostomy to the nonrefluxing ureter worked well in one patient, although the refluxing stump became a large diverticulum and was removed later. An attempt in another patient to reimplant only the refluxing ectopic ureter caused necrosis of both ureters and led ultimately to nephrectomy. The other six duplicated ureters were treated as if they were one within a common sheath and brought through a common tunnel; all these have worked well.

An early attempt at a Lich repair followed by a Hutch II resulted in atrophy of the kidney. However, there was severe ureteropyelocaliectasis and this kidney was probably salvable only by preliminary nephrostomy. None of the other 54 renal units operated on were dilated enough to require preliminary nephrostomy or tailoring to reduce ureteral caliber.

FOLLOW-UP COURSE

Voiding cystogram and intravenous pyelogram were performed approximately 3 months after surgery in 37 patients and will be done soon in two others. Cystoscopy was performed to assess anatomical result in some with normal X-rays and in all whose X-rays were not satisfactory. Urinalyses were performed monthly until clear. Antimicrobial drugs were given only for the 2 weeks after surgery, and as needed thereafter. The longest patient follow-up has been 10 years.

We have not advised repeated X-rays or cystoscopy for patients who no longer have reflux or damage to kidney or collecting system or who have not had recurrent urinary tract infections. However, such patients should have routine urinalysis at an established interval (3–6 months) and whenever symptoms or unexplained fevers occur.

RESULTS OF ANTIREFLUX SURGERY

Patients were classified as follows (Table 2): Good result (31 patients)—no reflux, pyelographic appearance as good or better than before operation, no recurrent clinical pyelonephritis. Acceptable result (four patients)—no recurrent pyelonephritis but stable minor pyelographic changes worse than before operation, no reflux. Bad result (two patients)—recurrent pyelonephritis, persistent obstruction or reflux, atrophy or loss of kidney. A "bad" rating could be temporary if subsequent surgery relieved obstruction (as in two patients now classified as "acceptable").

Unfavorable sequelae of operation are shown in Table 3. In four patients, contralateral reflux developed after unilateral reimplant; all have been managed conservatively thus far.

Table 2. Results of Antireflux Operation

	Children	Adults
Good	28	3
Acceptable	4	0
Bad	1	1
Not yet evaluated	2	0

Table 3. Unfavorable Sequelae of Antireflux Surgery

Persistent reflux, ultimate atrophy	1
Contralateral reflux	4
Ureteral necrosis, ultimate nephrectomy	1
Extramural obstruction, ureterolysis	1
Persistent anastomotic obstruction	1
Later Y-V plasty necessary	1
Recurrent cystitis	10

The ten patients who developed cystitis following complete recovery from reimplantation operation have been critically reviewed. None has had clinical pyelonephritis, reflux, or pyelographic change. Nearly all have a disordered micturition pattern, either infrequent voiding (three or four times a day) or frequency, urgency, and enuresis characteristic of the poorly inhibited bladder of childhood[5]. Infrequent voiders are asked to force fluids and void every 2–4 hr by the clock. Poorly inhibited bladders are treated with belladonna or imipramine.

Patients who give such hints of neurogenic bladder dysfunction should be treated appropriately before antireflux surgery is considered. If the renal condition nonetheless dictates operation, parents and physician should realize that correction of reflux may not prevent future cystitis but should confine infection to the bladder.

DISCUSSION

Successful nonoperative management of children with reflux depends upon vigilance of parents, pediatrician, and urologist. In 22% of our patients, antireflux surgery was necessary to preserve renal function, with 97% of them having a good or acceptable result (Table 2). These figures are similar to those of Nanninga et al.[6] and DeWeerd et al.[7], although our apparently better results are surely due to having only one patient with severe hydronephrosis when first seen. King et al[8]. have emphasized the poorer outcome of reimplantation in decompensated kidneys.

The four adults requiring nephrectomy for end-stage pyelonephritis and the 16 of 39 reimplanted patients whose kidneys were already damaged illustrate that some refluxing ureters must be reimplanted. But close observation has usually identified those needing intervention before occurrence of damage severe enough to prejudice the postoperative result. The series of Lyon et al[9]. emphasizes the value of careful follow-up, as 25 of his 67 patients reimplanted (37 %) required antireflux surgery 2 years or more after the first visit.

Our experience confirms the good results of reimplanting double ureters in their common sheath([10]) and the disastrous ischemic ureteral necrosis which can occur if they are separated.

REFERENCES

1. Creevy, C. D. Vesicoureteral reflux in children: A review. *Urol. Survey* **17**:279, 1967.
2. Spence, H. M. (moderator). Panel on ureteral reflux in children. *J. Urol.* **85**:119, 1961.
3. Graham, J. B., King, L. R., Kropp, K. A., and Uehling, D. T. The significance of distal urethral narrowing in young girls, *J. Urol.* **97**:1045, 1967.
4. Politano, V., and Leadbetter, W. F. An operative technique for the correction of vesicoureteral reflux. *J. Urol.* **79**:932, 1958.
5. Lapides, J., and Diokno, A. C. Persistence of the infant bladder as a cause for urinary infections in girls. *J. Urol.* **103**:243, 1970.
6. Nanninga, J., King, L. R., Downing, J., and Burden, J. J. Factors affecting the outcome of 100 reimplantations done for vesicoureteral reflux. *J. Urol.* **102**:772, 1969.
7. DeWeerd, J. H., Farsund, T., and Burke, E. C. Ureteroneocystostomy. *J. Urol.* **101**:520, 1969.
8. King, L. R., Surian, M. A., Wendel, R. M., and Burden, J. J. Vesicoureteral reflux. *J.A.M.A.* **203**:169, 1968.
9. Lyon, R. P., Marshall, S., and Tanagho, E. A. Theory of maturation: A critique. *J. Urol.* **103**:795, 1970.
10. Reule, G. R., and Ansell, J. S. Reimplantation of double ureters. J. *Urol.* **102**:172, 1969.

Studies on the Pathogenesis of Onchocerciasis

John A. C. Colston, Jr.*

Last winter it was my privilege to participate in a clinical investigation with the geographic epidemiology unit of Johns Hopkins University to study further the pathogenesis of onchocerciasis. The study took place in the Republic of Chad—formerly a part of French Equatorial Africa.

Onchocerciasis volvulus, also known as "river blindness," is carried by a filarial parasite and affects 30–40 million people in Central and East Africa and parts of Central America. It leads to blindness in 20% of its victims.

The adult worm is lodged in the subcutaneous tissue, where nodules are formed; microfilariae are discharged and transported via the lymphatic systems and presumably by this route enter the anterior chamber of the eye, leading to inflammation, sclerosis, and blindness. Microfilariae had been recovered from the urine sporadically in the past, but it was thought that they were harbored in the anterior urethra.

The principal focus of this investigation was to try to demonstrate the portal of entry into the urinary tract and the effect thereon of this disease. In a previous survey, onchocercal micofilaruria had been reported in 11% of the population of a small village of 200 inhabitants in Southern Chad named Ouli Bangala.

Our camp was set up on the Lim River close to this village. One hundred and fifty-three of the inhabitants (75%) were studied—this consisted of a physical examination, a *skin* survey by a dermatologist, an eye examination, etc. Routine urinalyses were done on all subjects, and when micro-

*The James Buchanan Brady Urological Institute, The Johns Hopkins Hospital, Baltimore, Maryland.

filariae were found, the individual, if he consented, was subjected to cystoscopy, bilateral ureteral catheterization, and retrograde pyelography. Twenty adults (11 females, nine males) including two controls were so studied.

On cystoscopy, the bladder mucosa was normal in all persons except one female who had early lesions of schistosomiasis hematobium confirmed by biopsy.

Therefore, from the cystoscopic findings there was no evidence to suggest that the primary portal of entry of the microfilariae into the urinary tract was the bladder. Living motile microfilariae were recovered from the renal pelvis via ureteral catheter in 45 % of the group. All microfilariae from the bladder urines were *dead*.

SPECIFIC FINDINGS ASSOCIATED WITH MICROFILARURIA

Fourteen pyelograms were readable. Four showed definite and similar ·radiographic findings: calyceal distortion–calyceal outlines lost. Fornices were blunted, compatible with chronic pyelonephritis and focal papillary necrosis.

There was albuminuria in most cases.

Blood pressure was normal.

With respect to renal function, all had normal blood urea nitrogen and creatinines. In general, those patients with microfilaruria had quantitatively heavier infections as indicated by *more* subcutaneous nodules and higher concentrations of microfilariae.

Malnutrition ranging from mild underweight to extreme cachexia was a constant finding. In these cases, tuberculosis was ruled out by chest X-rays.

Elevated serum glutamic oxalacetic transaminase (SGOT) was statistically significant and consistently higher in the microfilaruria group, indicating renal parenchymal damage.

CONCLUSIONS

These studies appear to demonstrate for the first time that microfilariae of onchocerciasis volvulus enter the urinary tract in the kidney, probably via pyelotubular lymphatics, and that the renal parenchyma is attacked directly, causing focal papillary necrosis.

Unfortunately, owing to the strong religious beliefs and the rigid burial customs of the Laka tribesmen, it is almost impossible to obtain histological confirmation of these clinical and radiological observations.

Recurrent Urethritis in the Female

William Nisbet Toole*

The female urethra is a short tube of relative anatomical simplicity (Fig. 1). Most urological textbooks, and even gynecological textbooks, treat this subject in a cursory manner. A search of the literature of the preantibiotic era produces a reasonable number of articles mainly dealing with that aspect of venereal disease affecting the female urethra. Nowadays, one sees a considerable amount written about pyelonephritis, the misuse of the catheter, and urinary tract bacteriology directed toward treatment with various drugs. There seems to be a lack of attention to anatomical pathology with respect to the epidemiology of urinary tract infections.

In my short span of practice, I have been deeply impressed by the number of females with recurrent urinary tract infections. By and large, these are females over 16 and under 60 years of age. (For purposes of this discussion, I am arbitrarily excluding the pediatric age group and the elderly.) Generally, by the time a patient reaches the urologist, she has had two or more bouts of cystourethritis. To my surprise, a considerable number of patients have been treated by other urologists and change physicians because of poor or short-term beneficial therapy. The following discussion is concerned with the anatomical basis of our program for treatment of this condition.

ANATOMY

The female urethra was the subject of two excellent papers by Huffman[1] and Krantz[2]. In these studies, the paraurethral glands were brought

*Department of Urology, Emory University School of Medicine, Atlanta, Georgia.

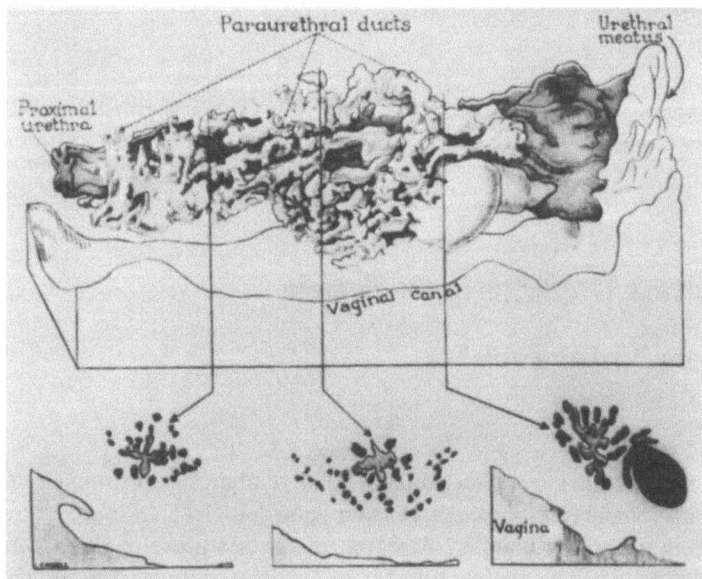

Fig. 1. Model of adult female urethra. Major number of complex ducts open into urethra just proximal to meatus. Small diagrams represent transverse section through urethra and glands.

into their true perspective. Although mentioned previously by Galen, de Graaf, Virchow, Oberdieck, Aschoff, Skene, and Hunner, the actual complexities of the paraurethral glands were finally shown and their pathophysiology explained.

Average length of most female urethras is 3–4 cm. When not dilated, the mucous membrane forms many longitudinal folds, causing the lumen to vary from from crescentic to stellate. The average caliber varies with age (see Table 1). At the external meatus, the epithelium is stratified squamous in type and progresses to pseudostratified in midurethra and transitional nearing the bladder neck.

The paraurethral glands surrounding the urethra take no particular pattern and are dispersed among the longitudinal muscle fibers. In the

Table 1. Average Caliber

Age	Caliber (F)
6 months	14
1 year	16
5 years	20
10 years	24
Adult	28

lower one-third they are not prominent, but often they extend the entire length of the urethra. Gland lining is simple columnar epithelium, and the gland type is simple tubular. Gland ducts are simple tubes opening directly into the urethra, except in the lower one-third, where some ducts may run parallel to the urethra and open on the vestibule at the external meatus. In Huffman's study, the number of paraurethral ducts varied from six to 31. Commonly, the two largest paraurethral glands are located at 5 and 7 o'clock and carry Skene's name because of his original description of their role in disease.

PATHOLOGY

The female urethra, unfortunately, opens into a moist, bacteria laden area. Because of this quirk of nature, the urethra is subjected to various forms of insult from infancy to senescence. These consist of fecal soilage, diaper irritations, masturbation, sexual relations, menstruation, vaginal, cervical, and uterine infections, and pregnancy, to name a few. Local trauma and the presence of bacteria produce an inflammatory response. The narrow duct orifices become occluded and lead to abscesses of varying sizes, usually draining through the urethra.

This process was proposed by Routh (1890) as the sequence of events in production of urethral diverticula. With repetition of this train of events over and over, the ducts cannot empty properly and carry a low-grade infection. The periurethral tissues become indurated and the urethral mucosa hyperemic and edematous. A coexistent cervicitis or vaginitis, or the edema associated with menstruation, makes matters worse. Sexual intercourse with this situation frequently triggers the subacute exacerbation of cystitis.

The observer examining such a patient can on stripping the urethra with his index finger express pus from the glands (Fig. 2). On examination of the distal urethra directly or the proximal urethra and bladder with the panendoscope, the urethral mucosa is seen to be injected and granular in appearance. The trigone often has a "cobblestone" appearance, and there are inflammatory polyps of the bladder neck tissue (Fig. 3) The bacteria on culture are usually Gram-negative rods, but may vary and are often seen mixed. I have yet to isolate *N. gonorrhea*. Not infrequently, when seen between exacerbations, the bladder on a catheterized urine specimen will be sterile, whereas the voided clean-catch urine or culture of the urethral strippings will show a high colony count.

SYMPTOMS

Women with chronic urethritis complain of urgency and frequency of urination. Frequently, they describe a "sticking" or burning sensation

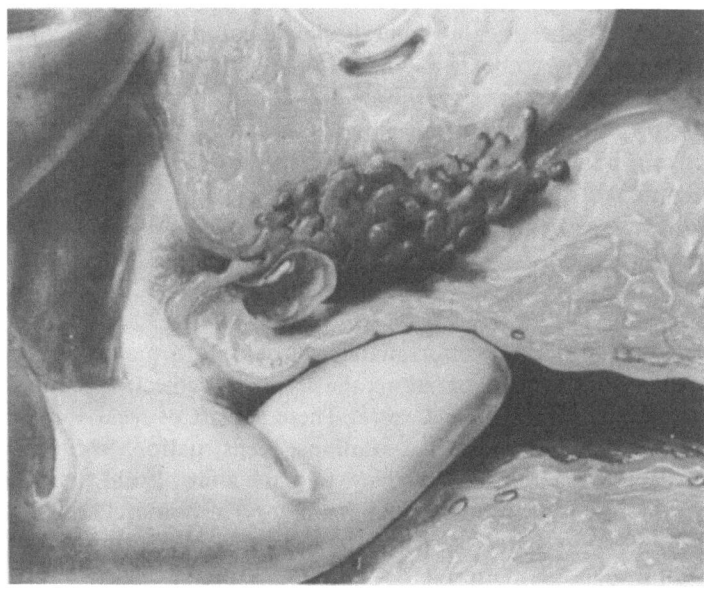

Fig. 2. Stripping the urethra to express the glands.

on voiding, and some have a constant dull lower pelvic discomfort. Often, they have referral of pain to the suprapubic area, lower back, or even higher in the abdomen. Dyspareunia is often present.

TREATMENT

The proper treatment of the woman with chronic or recurrent cysto-urethritis must begin with careful evaluation of the pathological conditions present. Direct visual examination of the distal one-thrid of the urethra and the external meatus can best be accomplished with the following instruments and light source: headlight, Mosher urethral speculum, plain tissue forceps, Bougie Thackston, Lacrimal duct probes (two), fine iris scissors, and Rieser electrode.

Urethral meatal stenosis of varying degrees, whether congenital or acquired, is frequently seen. Most of the patients whom we see with recurrent cystourethritis have at least one or more infected paraurethral glands, usually in the distal one-third of the urethra, which drain poorly and serve as constant reservoirs for reinfection. These can be detected with the small probe under direct vision (Fig. 4). The remainder of the urethra is best evaluated by using the MeCarthy panendoscope. If large infected glands are suspected in the proximal two-thirds of the urethra, a urethrogram should be made using the Davis–Cian catheter. I have located several totally unsuspected foci by this method.

After verification of the existing pathology, the proper treatment is then undertaken. Meatal stenosis is easily corrected by a midline meatotomy excising a sufficient wedge of the posterior urethral lip and suturing the mucosa with fine catgut sutures. If no large obstructed ducts are found, the urethra can be progressively dilated to promote emptying of the duct systems, as is common custom. However, urethral dilatation will not eradicate the obstructed duct system as a focus of infection, just as the use of antibacterial agents alone will not suffice. This has led us to the practice of unroofing the infected gland using a needle electrode and the high-frequency current of the Bovie electrosurgical unit (Fig. 5). It is impractical to excise most of these glands in the fashion one treats the urethral diverticulum because of their size and tendency to be multiple. Moreover, since most of the glands in question are in the distal one-third of the urethra, they are easily accessible. If there are larger glands higher in the urethra, these are

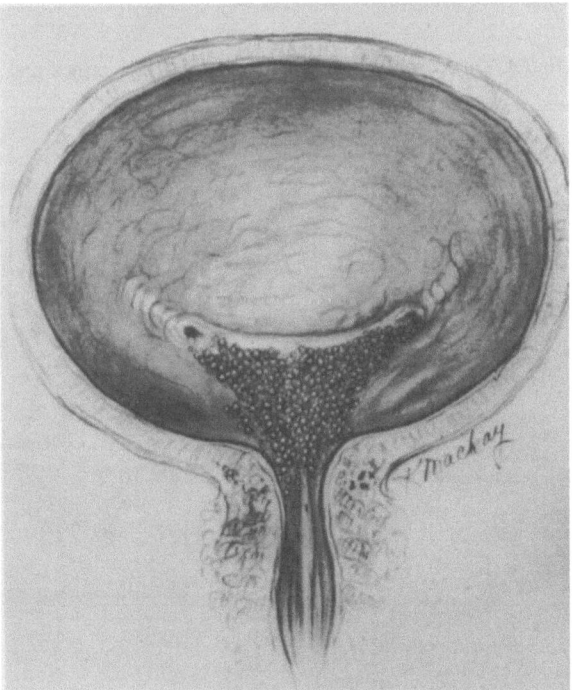

Fig. 3. Granular inflammatory changes seen on the
mucous membrane of the trigone.

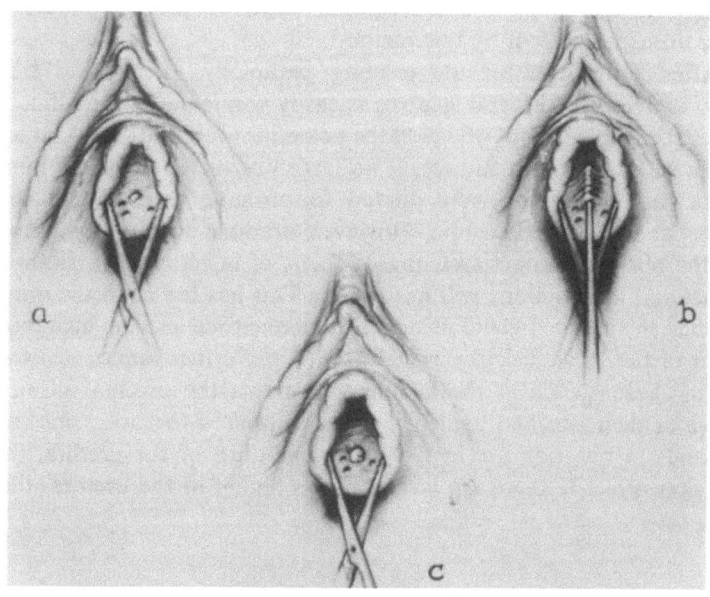

Fig. 4. Duct openings showing exudate at one orifice and
probe inserted in duct.

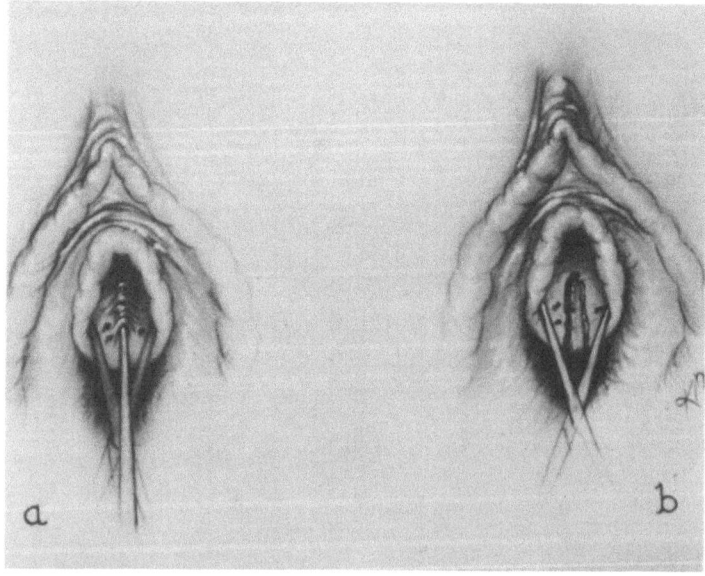

Fig. 5. Electrode in duct prior to unroofing and appearance after unroofing.

approached by a midline anterior vaginal incision. Inflammatory polyps of the bladder neck and the granular "cobblestone" mucosa of the bladder floor are usually "powder-burned" gently with the resectoscope. This seems to promote quicker healing and resolution of symptoms.

The bacterial infection is treated with the specific antibiotic according to culture results for 2 weeks, and the patient is maintained on supressive chemotherapy (sulfa, Furadantin) for 3 months. The patient is seen at routine intervals following surgery to evaluate healing of the urethra and general condition, i.e., 2 weeks, 6 weeks, and 12 weeks. At these times, we dilate the urethra to 34 F with Walther sounds. Generally, the bladder and urethra are well healed by the 12-week examination. Postoperative discomfort is usually over after the second week, or less in some patients. Following the 3-month visit, most patients no longer require any specific attention.

REFERENCES

1. Huffman, J. W. The detailed anatomy of the paraurethral ducts in the adult human female. *Amer. J. Obstet. Gynec.* **55**:86–100, 1648.
2. Krantz, K. E. The anatomy and physiology of micturition in the human female, read before the American Urological Association, New York, May 31, 1967.

HIGHLIGHTS

The Brady Urological Institute Origin, Growth, and Development

Hugh J. Jewett

In 1913 a momentous event occurred in American urology. Following a successful "punch operation" on James Buchanan Brady performed by Dr. Hugh Hampton Young, "Diamond Jim" agreed to donate funds to build and endow a urological institute at the Johns Hopkins Hospital, bearing his name in perpetuity. Up to this time, urological cases for the most part were scattered around the country throughout the wards of general surgery. Although surgeons relied at times on urologists for diagnosis, they reserved to themselves the right to operate whenever operation proved necessary. In most parts of the country, the urologists were not adequately trained as surgeons and their activities were limited to instrumentation and to the treatment of urinary infections and venereal disease. However, a few pioneers in urological surgery did exist, but they owed their distinction to the pleasure and generosity of their general surgical peers. Urology as a true specialty had not yet been born.

With the opening of the Brady Institute on January 21, 1915, a future for urology began to dawn. The building, affording facilities for patient care, teaching, and investigation, was the first of its kind in the Western Hemisphere. A chief of the service having lesser talents than those of Dr. Young might have muffed the extraordinary opportunity that was now promised. But Dr. Young proved to be just the right man at this auspicious moment.

The grandson and son of two generals in the Confederate Army, Dr. Young was born on September 18, 1870, His brilliant mind and high motivation enabled him to complete his undergraduate and medical education in record time, and after preliminary training in Baltimore he joined Dr.

William S. Halsted's surgical house staff in 1895. Two years later, at the age of 27, he was made chief of the Department of Genito-Urinary Diseases at the Johns Hopkins Hospital. His energy, native ability, curiosity, and leadership earned for him the rank of associate professor of urology in 1904. His ingenuity, dynamism, and fearlessness combined with technical skill soon placed him at the pinnacle of urological achievement in this country, and in 1914 he became clinical professor.

Dr. Young's assumption of control of the new Brady Institute in 1915 marked the beginning of an extraordinarily productive era during which the infant specialty of urology began to thrive. He trained 38 residents, of whom 11 became chiefs of urological services in other university centers. In addition to acquiring a large and lucrative clinical practice, he published 350 original articles and three textbooks, and became editor of *The Journal of Urology* which he founded. In the period between the two World Wars the Brady Institute was virtually seething with activity, and as a world-renowned center of first-class urological diagnosis and surgery, attracted numerous postgraduate students and observers from this country and from abroad.

Dr. Young retired in 1942 at the age of 71. Dr. J. A. Campbell Colston then became acting chief of the service, pending the appointment of a new professor. Dr. Colston, thoroughly competent, warm, and human, steeped in the best traditions of the Brady, served with distinction for 4 years. He then, in accordance with the prearranged plan, was asked in 1946 to step down and hand over the reins of authority to Dr. William Wallace Scott.

It was into this established urological environment of international renown that Dr. Scott, fresh from the University of Chicago, found himself suddenly immersed in October of that year at the age of 33. Throughout the country the eyes of his medical peers were on him. Could he handle the job? Would he muddle through? Could he attract another benefactor like Diamond Jim? Would he eventually become a vital force in American urology?

Dr. Scott was unperturbed. He knew that diagnostic and surgical urology had progressed to a remarkable extent, but believed that the time had come to develop the clinical specialty into a solid structure with roots sunk deep in the basic sciences. Earlier he had purposely interrupted his medical school career for two years to earn a Ph. D. degree in physiology. After obtaining his degree in medicine he continued to pursue his interests in the laboratory. He came to the Brady Institute not only with the necessary clinical skills, but also with a keen mind trained in laboratory medicine. With the whole hearted cooperation of the Johns Hopkins School of Medicine and Hospital he redesigned and renovated the top floor of the Brady Institute for laboratory research and obtained funds for the required personnel, apparatus, and animals.

This laboratory has served as a training ground for assistant residents who, under expert guidance, have been introduced to original investigative techniques, and taught to think for themselves. No pronouncements by distinguished physicians are held sacred by authority alone, but must stand on their own merits in the light of penetrating analysis. The healthy effect of such teaching and influence has resulted in renewed attention to the Brady Institute, from which seven of Dr. Scott's residents have become full professors in university centers, and five others are chiefs of service. The distinction of the service has also been reflected in the high quality of the men seeking appointment to the residency training program after having finished their two years in general surgery.

In contrast to the interests of his predecessor, Dr. Scott has succeeded in interweaving policy and administration with that of the university and hospital and has served on ten important committees of the school of medicine. His professional performance as head of the Brady Institute during the last quarter-century has been extraordinarily productive. In a quiet, unassuming manner he has earned for himself and for his service the high regard and respect of all levels of medical science in and out of government, at home and abroad.

The Brady Institute, during his tenure, has been not only viable but truly progressive. In 25 years, endowment funds have grown, training and project grants have been obtained, and 431 papers have been published. The Institute is still in the forefront of American Urology, and under such enlightened leadership seems destined to remain there.

Dr. William W. Scott's 25th Anniversary at Johns Hopkins

Clarence Hodges*

January 1, 1971, will mark my 30 years of association with Professor William Wallace Scott in pursuits related to Urology. The setting was the laboratory of Dr. Charles B. Huggins at the University of Chicago where I had spent my senior elective quarter. Having graduated in December, 1940, I continued to work as a research fellow on the use of serum phosphatases as an indicator when hormonal control of prostatic cancer was instituted. Dr. Huggins was Professor and Chief of the Division of Urology and Dr. Cornelius Vermeulen was an Instructor in Urology. Dr. Scott came to the laboratory, having just completed a year of straight surgical internship, to spend six months in research prior to entering the residency program in Urology.

Bill Scott had taken time out, as many did at the University of Chicago, to obtain a Ph.D. in Physiology between his second and third years of medical school. He had worked under such giants as Professors Anton J. Carlson and Arno B. Luckhardt in the Department of Physiology, elucidating the mechanism of the knockout blow in boxing. Their influence was apparent in his logical approach to an experimental problem and his insistence on scientific evidence for any conclusions drawn. He set up a study for estimation of acid and alkaline phosphatases in urine and had all of us in the laboratory contributing 24-hr specimens. With the help of his father's exquisite gold pocket watch and Dr. Huggins' slide rule, Bill and I were able to run serum or urine phosphatase determinations in batches of 100 to 150 in a half day doing the final steps in the King–Armstrong method at the rate of one every 15 seconds.

*University of Oregon School of Medicine, Dept. of Urology, Portland, Oregon.

A very complicated combination of glassware formed a still which Professor Frederick Koch (Biochemistry) had used in his early epochal work on steroid hormones. This was made available to Bill for further studies on isolation of hormones from urine. Necessary repairs were obtained through the services of a talented glassblower in the Physics Department. It required two of us to carry the equipment to the Physics Building and subsequently, in its fragile completed form, back to our laboratory. We had it beautifully set up and ready to try out when Dr. Huggins walked in whistling some nameless tune—the apparatus promptly cracked. We sadly carried it back to the glassblower who carefully and skillfully repaired it again. We joyfully carried it back to the laboratory, set it up again, Dr. Huggins walked in whistling the same tune and it cracked again! After the third repair, the apparatus was successfully installed and functioned well thereafter (perhaps Dr. Huggins changed his tune).

In June, 1941, we (Doctors Huggins, Gomori, Scott, and I) presented an exhibit on "Prostatic Cancer: Hormonal Influences" at the Annual American Medical Association meeting in Cleveland. Exhibits were not so complex in those days and this one could be easily strapped to the top of Bill's old green 1935 Chevrolet. This was a wonderful car; Bill was very generous in lending it, and it had provided the setting for several house officer romances and at least two couples had taken it on their honeymoon. On this occasion, Bill and I drove to Cleveland with the exhibit while Doctors Huggins and Gomori took the train. This remarkable car had only one indubitable weakness at that point; without warning, the hood would fly up, completely ruling out forward vision! This helped to keep both driver and passenger awake.

An interesting sidelight, the University of Chicago advanced 100 dollars which was ample for the expenses of the four of us for travel and living expenses during the five-day convention.

After World War II, I resumed the Urology residency at the University of Chicago where Bill Scott was now Assistant Professor. He was always very generous with his time, both as a teacher and as a friend. When Dr. Huggins decided to accept the position of Professor of Urology at Johns Hopkins University and Hospital, following the death of Hugh Young in 1945, Dr. Scott was appointed Professor of Urology at the University of Chicago. Subsequently, Dr. Huggins decided to remain at the University of Chicago and Bill's future seemed uncertain. He allowed the University of Chicago to cancel his hardly dry contract as Professor of Urology and considered a part-time appointment at the University of Illinois. This restless period was terminated when Dr. Alfred Blalock offered Bill the position at Hopkins which Dr. Huggins had renounced. During this period, Bill made it possible for me to enter the Johns Hopkins rotation by spending most of the year with Dr. Fred Foley at Anchor Hospital and going on to Johns Hopkins for a final year of residency in Baltimore. These had been the sixth and seventh years of the residency program developed by Dr. Hugh Young. The details of Bill's early years at Hopkins, the setting up of the experimental laboratories, and the continued outstanding quality of the Hopkins Residency in Urology will undoubtedly be portrayed by others.

During these more than 30 years, Bill's influence in relating basic science to Urology, his insistence on scientific documentation of discovery, his tremendous capacity for hard work, and his stimulating example to others have been most beneficial to Urology. As always, behind every great man there is a great woman—in this case, the lovely, charming, and wonderful Jessie Lou has helped to make all this possible.

Reminiscences

From The Urological Residency at Johns Hopkins (by David M. Davis)

...A few years ago I wrote in an essay on *Forty Years of Urology in Retrospect* the following: "Clinical research must include determination of the best methods of application directly to the patient, and must not neglect considerations of safety. In some instances, it must provide the whole answer to the question posed, but in others, it must seek more widely afield and so act as a bridge between fundamental research and the patient. It is a pity that a good many young men have come to feel a little contemptuous of clinical research, and that in order to prove superior intellectual capacity, they must engage in something which is, or at least seems to approach, fundamental research. Good clinical research requires a keen and active brain, a wide range of knowledge, and a complete dissatisfaction with the orthodox and the routine. It has need of many active and competent practitioners."

These views appear to have gained confirmation during the years of Dr. Scott's leadership. In the face of the great changes which have taken place, the financial difficulties, the invasion, further and further, of government and politics into medicine, the Brady has kept on toward the goals set for it at its founding, the validity of which has only become clearer as the years have passed.

It is indeed a pleasure and a privilege to take part in this well-earned recognition of Dr. Scott's great services—to the Brady, to the Hopkins, to medicine by his teaching and by his research programs and accomplishments; and to the great army of the sick and troubled.

From a Letter to William Wallace Scott from Ormond S. Culp

Although I belong to an older vintage of "Brady Boys," you have my heartiest congratulations and profound admiration on the Silver Anniversary of your Brady Directorship. This occasion must not pass without my testimony even though I did not have the privilege of working under you and had to settle for H.H.Y.

All of us "old-timers" know how difficult it was to succeed "The Professor." You accomplished the feat with so much distinction during the past 25 years that we are truly proud of your record. You have added to the glamour, traditions, and reputation of the Brady. I am sure that former residents are most grateful and have enjoyed basking in the reflected glory....

I can appreciate what your personal protégés feel because you have had a great impact on all of Urology. Contemporaries, as well as residents, have become more knowledgeable because of your scientific talents, personality, and superb communication.... May your next 25 years be equally exciting, stimulating, and productive!

The Professor (by H. John Bradley, Jr.)

How can you adequately honor a man of deeds with mere words. Dr. William Wallace Scott is recognized throughout the scientific world for his research, teaching, and editing in the field of Urology. This says nothing of his contributions as author, surgeon, and administrator. His students, residents, fellows, and associates are literally scattered over the entire free world. Their accomplishments and activities reflect the quality of their training at the Brady Urologic Institute. The many prestigeous positions occupied by these men attest to Dr. Scott's ability to select and inspire men of talent.

After much consideration I have decided that only some positive presentation would honor a man of this nature. His interest and research into the problem of prostatic cancer has not resulted in a cure for this dread disease, however, we have learned much over the past twenty-five years that has contributed to the control of this malignancy. Dr. Scott could have selected many easier problems which would have resulted in greater personal satisfaction and professional advancement, but this was not his way. His unofficial motto always being, "We work hard, we play hard, and when the going gets rough we don't put in a good eight hours, but we put in twelve or eighteen hours or whatever it takes to solve the problem."

From the scientific point of view I wish this was a large series, but all series are made up of case reports. All case reports are but brief outlines of the real people who live, suffer, and die under our care. There can be no greater satisfaction for the physician than to say, "I have helped this man."

No greater tribute can be paid to Dr. Scott than to recall the thousands of patients who have benefited from his interest and insistence that we apply the scientific method to the practice of medicine.

One day when I was Assistant Resident on the Private Service, Dr. Colston, Sr., was recalling those difficult first few months after Dr. Scott took over the Brady Urological Institue. He mentioned the many dificult decisions and problems which faced Dr. Scott, but what impressed me most was that he said throughout this diffucult time he (Dr. Scott) was always a gentleman. To those of us who have been privileged to work closely with him and receive our training under his guidance he has given a special meaning to the title of the Professor.

From a Letter to William Wallace Scott from Kenneth Walton

...For me the years at Hopkins are wonderful memories and where I have four, you have twenty-five. Through those that trained there you have influenced the care of many patients. Many of the residents have since helped educate other students and residents. Sometimes we little realize our influence. On this twenty-fifth anniversary we, the "old boys" ask you to reflect a moment. As you sit by the fireplace, perhaps pat the dog, and muse over times past, smile, Professor, for you and the Johns Hopkins Hospital were the reasons we came.

A Word from California—In Thanks to William Wallace Scott from John A. Arcadi

Accolades to Dr. William Wallace Scott from a urologist practicing in a little town in the West seem anticlimactic and very inadequate. But to Bill Scott, my friend, I say thanks—thanks for so many things that I dare not try to enumerate here. To relate my first and earliest associations with Bill Scott is the purpose of this discourse, to show his concern for an individual—an example of his overall concern for those of us who have had the privilege to have him as our mentor....

It was apparent to me, by 1948, that urology was my ultimate goal and doing research in that or related fields was very important to me particularly if it could be under the direction of Bill Scott. I spent as much time as possible in the Brady Urological Dispensary, doing circumcisions, seeing patients, and watching experts do cystoscopies.

Dr. William Wallace Scott, whom we love and honor this day, was, and is, a man to be seen and listened to—a man who gave of himself to any problem of the medical student.

By late 1949, when it was time to apply for internships at the Hopkins, I applied to Dr. Richard TeLinde in Gynecology and to Dr. Scott in Urology. As early spring 1950 arrived, I heard a rumor that Dr. TeLinde had accepted me as an intern in his department, but no word had leaked out about my prime choice, my great academic desire—to be a Brady intern.

A few days later—it seems like weeks or months—I was standing in the elevator lobby of Halsted waiting to go up to my surgical floor when Dr. Scott came off the elevator. I recall that moment well. He looked directly at me and said, "You're Johnny Arcadi, aren't you?" in that voice that I have come to know, love, and imitate over these twenty years. I replied I was, in a quavering voice, and he said, "I understand you would like to be an intern in urology. Well, I know your record and your interest and you have the job—if you want it." Did I want it—WOW! I thanked him profusely and my life reached heights I had only dreamed of.

Bill Scott affected me most on two occasions in the following year and a half in my internship. It was at the end of our year of internship in the spring of 1951. Others apparently had been selected to stay on at the Brady, but above all, I wanted to stay at least another year but in the research laboratory. The Professor and I talked in his office about my future. He knew of my great desire to spend a year doing research in *his* laboratory. He, after seemingly exploring his being, told me I could work in the laboratory for a year—but with no assurance of going on through the residency. I was in the department of a great man and I knew it! Further plans were subjugated to my subconscious.

When my year in the lab was coming to a close, the Professor shocked me in his inimitable way. At our morning coffee break in April or early May of 1952, Bill Scott said, "Johnny, now would you like to go to Shelbyville and come back here for the residency?" Would I? Yes, indeed! How fortunate can a man be when he's young, doing the things he wants to do at the place he wants to be, under a man he admires and respects?

Bill made a statement that really sums up the aim and purpose of the Brady Residency better than I—"I can teach you all the operations in urology in a week, but when to operate, when not to operate, and what to do in times of trouble will take at least five years to learn."

Since leaving the Brady in 1955, my life has been good. I enjoy doing clinical urology and especially basic research. So, thank you, Bill Scott. I have learned well from you.

William Wallace Scott's First Days at The Brady

During the annual session of the American College of Surgeons in Chicago, October 14, 1970, Herbert Brendler, Willard E. Goodwin, Peter L. Scardino, and Perry B. Hudson met at the Palmer House, to record vignettes that touched on the first days of W. W. Scott at Johns Hopkins. Three were house officers at the Brady Urological Institute when Dr. Scott arrived in October 6, 1946. Dr. Hudson was Dr. Scott's first appointment to the house staff to replace C. V. Hodges. A recording was made of the meeting of the four former house officers. Below are some excerpts from this meeting.

P.S.: In late 1945 I went to Baltimore for an interview at The Johns Hopkins Hospital. The first person I met after Dr. Colston was a Dr. Brendler.

H.B.: Well, on with it, what did I do?

P.S.: Do you remember on Brady 3, greeting me with George Strong who was leaving to go to Philadelphia? After Dr. Colston introduced me to Herb, he invited me to put on a well-powdered glove to examine a patient with prostatic carcinoma. The powder covered my navy blue uniform, which convulsed Herb and the retinue of house officers. After I brushed myself clean, Dr. Colston took me to meet the famous Dr. Blalock. We went toward the hospital dining room, it now being one o'clock. Outside the big swinging doors we met the renowned heart surgeon. Quite humbly, I thought, Dr. Colston stopped Dr. Blalock to ask: "Al, I have a young Naval officer who wants to be an intern in Urology. Is it all right with you if I give him the job?" Blalock replied, "Well Cap, whatever you want is all right with me." Sometime later the *New York Times* carried a picture of Dr. Charles Huggins, the new Professor of Urology at the Johns Hopkins.

H.B.: When did you see that in the newspaper?

P.S.: Now this I can't remember, but it was after my trip to Baltimore in the winter of 1945–46.

W.G.: I got out of the Army in the Fall of that year. I worked in Dr. Blalock's department for a while. It became known somehow that Dr. Huggins was going to the Professor. I had never met Dr. Huggins He was a friend of my Uncle Elmer. I didn't want to be left off the list. Dr. Huggins would come with about twenty assistant

215

residents from Chicago. I wrote Dr. Huggins that I was here and wanted to see him when he came. As a matter of fact he had already been and was coming back. I met him on a Sunday afternoon. He said he wanted to see Baltimore. I drove him around town and to the edge of an estuary where the ships dock in the middle of Baltimore. It was a bitter March day; the wind was blowing; it was slightly raining; the trees hadn't gotten green yet. It was cold and miserable. "Look," I said, "see the Baltimore harbor." Dr. Huggins looked at it. His only reply was: "Will, it is a *bleak prospect.*" It was a great deal later that I learned that someone else was coming to be the Professor.

H.B.:   I can remember at some point on Brady 1, someone asked Hugh Jewett what was going on. He said, "Doggonest thing." We asked him what he wanted to do with all the slides that were on file. He said, "just throw them out." Dr. Young had accumulated those things for years. The whole Brady is bound up in those gross specimens down in the basement and all these slides that Slade has been filing. He said, "just throw them out." Can you imagine that?

P.S.:   Jewett said that?

H.B.:   What was it like to be young, partly-trained, uneasy, and expecting a new Professor after the death of Hugh Hampton Young and the regrets of Dr. Huggins?

P.S.:   I remember well the atmosphere of tension. Would we be allowed to stay and finish the residency; Cap and Blalock had made the appointments. Would we be allowed to serve it out? There was, I think, understandable nervousness about Dr. Scott coming to the Brady, not only because he was a new broom, but because of the people he would bring and appoint to insert into the program and perhaps delay our completing the Hopkins experience. After four years of life on shipboard and in Navy installations, the 8–4 existence of a bureaucrat, more lieutenant than doctor, more scuttlebutt than fact, more fiction than science, it was incredible how genuinely united all the Brady staff was behind this young man. Everyone was pulling for him; everyone was behind him; I do not remember one time in his first three years there when there was any gossip or criticism socially, or among the wives. I wonder if Bill knew that? It was unique in my experience, such loyalty.

. . . .

W.G.:   The other memory I had is of one day Dr. Huggins came to make rounds with Dr. Colston. The Cap was head of the service. Dr. Colston introduced the residents to the new Professor. "Gentlemen," he said, "I want you to meet Dr. Higgins." Dr. Huggins said in a quite loud voice, "Huggins is the name. Huggins, *not* Higgins!"

H.B.:   I remember the day Dr. Scott arrived, I was on duty. He called on a Sunday night. I was the resident; Evan Lewis, the intern, was on with me. We had a man who had pushed a pencil up his urethra. We were debating what to do about it. We had the bladder open, there was the pencil. You could see it in the bladder. You could feel it in the urethra; he pushed it in point first, of course. We were talking about this and debating whether we would have to break the pencil in the perineum or just how to work this thing out. A phone message came that *a* Dr. Scott had called. This was about 8:00 P.M. They informed us that this was *the* Dr. Scott. We dealt with the pencil. I went out and called Dr. Scott. This was the first time I had ever spoken with him. He said, "Herb, this is Bill Scott. I am here at Dr. Blalock's house. I am all alone." I asked where the Blalocks were? "Well, they have all gone. He is going to let me stay here because I don't have any place to stay. My wife and little boy are in Chicago, and, Herb, I'm lonely." That's just exactly what happened. I told him we had just finished a case and had not had dinner. I remember Maggie and I took Bill Scott to a Chinese restaurant (Jimmy Wu's on North Charles Street).

This was my first contact with him. That was October 7, 1946.

P.S.: You know Perry was almost too much for Dr. Scott that's why Perry fired him. Do you remember the night you fired Dr. Scott, Perry?

P.H.: No.

P.S.: You don't? Well, *he* does, he has told me about it.

P.H.: No, while you guys were doing all this, I was on my way back from Shanghai. It really is funny to sit here in Chicago and think back more than thirty years when I was here in this city as a graduate student. I didn't know either Dr. Scott or Dr. Huggins. This was before Dr. Huggins had published his work on prostatic cancer for which he won the Nobel prize in medicine. It is kind of weird that the footprints go around from one institution to another. To see Dr. Huggins and then Dr. Scott. come from here, the University of Chicago, to Baltimore.

P.H.: I suppose the only bridge however, between Hugh Young Urology and Scott Urology is you, Will. Obviously you are the only one that went to school at Hopkins, interned and then came back. You always seemed more Johns Hopkins than Johns Hopkins. I remember coming right after Dr. Scott came and the first person I saw when I got there was Herb Brendler. I came quite by accident to visit Justina Hill, Dr. Young's bacteriologist and an old family friend. She introduced me to Dr. Scott. He said, "If you don't like where you are now working, why not work here?" When I implied that I preferred working in a laboratory, he warmed immediately and suggested that he could possibly make such an arrangement.

. . . .

W.G.: I had some feelings about Dr. Scott and his early days at Hopkins. Having been on the scene, and having a vested interest in what was going to happen, I couldn't afford to be antagonistic. At the same time I had a feeling of reserve. What are we going to get? But it didn't take me very long to accept that here was a leader who I could follow with pleasure. Although I didn't agree with everything he had to say or even feel, he knew more than I did about some things.

. . . .

P.H.: You know, I had more arguments with Dr. Scott I bet, than all you guys put together. I remember the time he fired me. We had a lot of arguments. I never really disagreed in terms of the purposes he had in mind. I never did think he changed those. When you said what you did about the Johns Hopkins, I think a lot of people feel that way about it and about him. After I got to New York at the age of 32, and tried to put together a residency program and a laboratory of my own, I began to think back what it must have been like for this man coming into those circumstances. I was at Columbia when things were hard, and anything you did that was good would be an advance. He came into an institute that was widely known all over the world in terms of its Professors. In fact, the Professor who preceded him was the world's greatest urologist. So the circumstances were different. Yet, I found it hard enough in New York. Then I began to rethink a lot about this stuff, It will shock everybody, but the ideals were involved, the idealism that was involved in his coming there and doing what he did, maybe was tempered sometimes and maybe not, but with consistency. That really was where the payoff was and I thought in those days, and I think today, that how you do it is not so important, as what it is that you're doing, and why you're doing it too. Because how you will do it, is really a function of personality.

. . . .

W.G.: Well, you have made a great statement for all of us. It's sort of the way Dr. Blalock's residents feel about him. Because they say the same sort of things; you don't understand him but you appreciate him. And I would think that maybe, what would be important to me is that I wouldn't be where I am in Urology today if I hadn't had this stimulus to my environment. It wasn't always the stimulus that I liked, but maybe that's important. To have something to make you move. I think the thing he gave to me, above everything else, was the chance to work in his lab, and the chance to have his support in whatever I could get from him talking to him, but also the chance for a free hand to do whatever I wanted to. This made a big impression on me, it really did. We weren't that much separated in years, but he was sort of a father image; to say, "well O.K. lad go ahead and do this, but come talk to me if you want some advice." I suppose that that meant more to me than anything else at that time in my life, and in my future career, to have that kind of an experience. I'm not trying to sell it to anybody, but that's what I got out of it.

Author Index

Acardi, J. A., 211
Aliapoulios, M. A., 25
Bradley, H. J., Jr., 210
Brannan, W., 69
Brendler, H., 61, 215
Carter, M. F., 27
Chung, L. W. K., 27
Coffey, D. S., 27
Colston, J. A. C., Jr., 189
Culp, O. S., 210
Davis, D. M., 119, 209
DeKlerk, J. N., 51
Engel, R. M., 169
Goodwin, W. E., 75, 215
Grayhack, J. T., 39
Hodges, C., 205
Holland, J. M., 181
Hudson, P. B., 215
Huggins, C. B., 3
Jewett, H. J., 201

King, L. R., 89
Leiter, E., 151
Maguire, J. W., 61
Mirand, E. A., 123
Mittelman, A., 161
Murphy, G. P., 123
Persky, L., 81
Scardino, P. L., 215
Schirmer, H. K. A., 157
Schmidt, J. D., 107
Schwartz, H., 173
Scott, W. W., 3, 7, 21, 27, 28, 39, 75, 89,
    107, 129, 131, 157, 169, 173, 202, 203,
    205, 207, 209–211, 215
Silk, M., 21
Stamey, T. A., 131
Toole, W. N., 191
Walton, K. N., 211
Williams-Ashman, H. G., 7
Young, H. H., 201, 202

Subject Index

Amino acid, 9, 16, 17, 18
Androgen, 8, 25, 26, 27
Angiography, 61, 65, 66
Anomaly, 61, 117, 146, 151, 169
Anti-androgen, 27, 30, 31, 42, 45
Antibiotic, 173, 179
Antibody, 21, 23, 178

Bacteria, 173, 175
Biochemistry, 4
Bladder, 51, 52, 56, 59, 76, 142, 181
Brady Urological Institute, 201, 205, 209–213, 215

Calculi, 103, 108
Cancer, 3, 22, 28, 29, 65
Canine, 25, 39, 43, 69
Carcinogens, 3, 4
Castrate, 29, 32, 45
Citric acid, 43, 44
Colon, 76, 78
Cystocele, 52
Cystogram, 55

Diethylstilbestrol, 22, 23
Diverticula, 54
DMBA, 4, 5
DNA, 8, 28, 29, 30, 32, 35, 37

Enzyme, 15
Erythropoietin, 123, 126–129
Estrogen, 21, 22, 28, 29, 32, 33, 42

Fructose, 43

Gel-diffusion, 44

Horseshoe kidney, 146, 153, 154
Human, 25
Hydrocarbon, 3
Hydronephrosis, 101, 160
Hyperplasia, 28, 29, 39, 41, 43, 47
Hypertension, 125, 126, 131, 139
Hypophysectomy, 29, 44
Hypospadias, 169
Hysterectomy, 52, 72

Ileum, 76, 77, 81, 84, 85, 89, 90, 93, 97, 99, 107, 108, 112, 113, 117
Intestine, 75, 77
Ischemia, 131, 142, 157

Jejunum, 101

Kidney, 61, 62, 65, 66, 73, 124, 125, 134,
    144, 146, 151, 157

L-Isomer, 10, 11, 18
L-Ornithine, 10

Mammalian, 10
Metabolism, 157
Methionine, 16
Methylthioadenosine, 15
Micturition, 55

Nephrectomy, 63, 64
Nephrostomy, 70, 101, 103, 104, 117
Nonandrogenic, 43
Nuclei, 31

Onochocerciasia, 189
Operation, 57, 58
Orchiectomy, 17, 30, 42
Oxygen, 158

Pelvis, 51, 52
Plasma, 23
Polyamines, 7, 16
Progestins, 42
Prostate, 7, 17, 22, 25, 26, 27, 29, 31, 37,
    39, 41, 45,
Protein, 17, 23, 29
Psychosomatic, 59, 60
Putrasine, 8, 10

Radiation, 116
Rat, 3, 30, 43, 46, 160, 167
Reflux, 181, 186, 187

Renin, 123, 126–129, 131, 133
RNA, 29, 30, 32

Seminal vesicle, 27, 43, 44
Spermidine, 8, 10, 14
Spermine, 8, 10, 15
Steroid, 25, 135, 139
Stilbestrol, 21
Stoma, 81, 82, 86, 87, 91, 108–110
Synthesis, 17

Teflon, 31
Testis, 44, 45, 133
Testosterone, 25, 26, 31, 35, 40, 41, 43, 44

Uremia, 103, 119, 120, 123, 125, 126, 160
Ureter, 69, 70, 73, 76, 78, 81, 90, 91, 94,
    95, 98, 99, 104, 112
Urethra, 52, 191, 192
Urethritis, 191
Urine, 43, 44, 109, 133, 172, 173

Ventral prostate, 17, 28, 32, 43
Veteran's group, 21

Wet weight, 43
Wound, 116

Xylene, 31

Yeast, 165

Zess, 128